James C. Fisher
Henry C. Simmons

A Journey Called Aging
Challenges and Opportunities in Older Adulthood

NOTES FOR PROFESSIONAL LIBRARIANS AND LIBRARY USERS

This is an original book title published by The Haworth Press, Taylor & Francis Group. Unless otherwise noted in specific chapters with attribution, materials in this book have not been previously published elsewhere in any format or language.

CONSERVATION AND PRESERVATION NOTES

All books published by The Haworth Press and its imprints are printed on certified pH neutral, acid-free book grade paper. This paper meets the minimum requirements of American National Standard for Information Sciences-Permanence of Paper for Printed Material, ANSI Z39.48-1984.

DIGITAL OBJECT IDENTIFIER (DOI) LINKING

The Haworth Press is participating in reference linking for elements of our original books. (For more information on reference linking initiatives, please consult the CrossRef Web site at www.crossref.org.) When citing an element of this book such as a chapter, include the element's Digital Object Identifier (DOI) as the last item of the reference. A Digital Object Identifier is a persistent, authoritative, and unique identifier that a publisher assigns to each element of a book. Because of its persistence, DOIs will enable The Haworth Press and other publishers to link to the element referenced, and the link will not break over time. This will be a great resource in scholarly research.

A Journey Called Aging

Challenges and Opportunities in Older Adulthood

THE HAWORTH PRESS

Rev. James W. Ellor, DMin, DCSW, CGP
Melvin A. Kimble, PhD
Co-Editors in Chief

A Journey Called Aging
Challenges and Opportunities in Older Adulthood

James C. Fisher
Henry C. Simmons

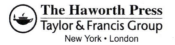
The Haworth Press
Taylor & Francis Group
New York • London

BP53

For more information on this book or to order, visit
http://www.haworthpress.com/store/product.asp?sku=5915

or call 1-800-HAWORTH (800-429-6784) in the United States and Canada
or (607) 722-5857 outside the United States and Canada
or contact orders@HaworthPress.com

The Haworth Press, Taylor & Francis Group, 270 Madison Avenue, New York, NY 10016.

PUBLISHER'S NOTE

The development, preparation, and publication of this work has been undertaken with great care. However, the Publisher, employees, editors, and agents of The Haworth Press are not responsible for any errors contained herein or for consequences that may ensue from use of materials or information contained in this work. The Haworth Press is committed to the dissemination of ideas and information according to the highest standards of intellectual freedom and the free exchange of ideas. Statements made and opinions expressed in this publication do not necessarily reflect the views of the Publisher, Directors, management, or staff of The Haworth Press, or an endorsement by them.

Excerpt from "Do Not Go Gentle Into That Good Night," by Dylan Thomas, from THE POEMS OF DYLAN THOMAS, copyright © 1952 by Dylan Thomas. Reprinted by permission of New Directions Publishing Corp.
    Sales Territory: U.S./Canadian rights only. For all other territories refer to: David Higham Associates, Ltd., 5-8 Lower John St., Golden Square, London W1R 4HA, ENGLAND. Tel. 44 207 437 7888; Fax. 44 207 437 1072.

Cover design by Kerry E. Mack.

Library of Congress Cataloging-in-Publication Data

Fisher, James C.
    A journey called aging : challenges and opportunities in older adulthood / James C. Fisher, Henry C. Simmons.
        p. cm.
    Includes bibliographical references.
    ISBN: 978-0-7890-3383-3 (hard : alk. paper)
    ISBN: 978-0-7890-3384-0 (soft : alk. paper)
    1. Older people—Social conditions. 2. Older people—Psychology. 3. Aging. 4. Old age.
I. Simmons, Henry C. II. Title.

HQ1061.F53 2007
305.26—dc22

                                                                                2007000547

4/30/09

To our wives, Barbara Cech Fisher
and Helen Cecile McDonald,
as we travel together
on the journey called aging

ABOUT THE AUTHORS

James C. Fisher, PhD, is Associate Professor of Adult and Continuing Education Emeritus at the University of Wisconsin-Milwaukee, where he has been a faculty member since 1981. He is an ordained minister in the Presbyterian Church and currently serves as Parish Associate at Immanuel Presbyterian Church, Milwaukee. His major interests are in older adult development, learning, and educational activities. Dr. Fisher has served on the boards of directors of Carroll College and Literacy Services of Wisconsin. His publications include *The Welfare-to-Work Challenge for Adult Literacy Educators* (with Larry G. Martin), *Using Learning to Meet the Challenges of Older Adulthood* (with Mary Alice Wolf), and *Leadership and Management of Volunteer Programs* (with Kathleen M. Cole).

Henry C. Simmons, PhD, is Professor of Religion and Aging at Union Theological Seminary and Presbyterian School of Education, where he has taught since 1985. His major interests include the spiritual growth of older adults, ethics and aging, congregational studies, and ecology and religion. He is an ordained minister and is active in several community service organizations, including the Fan Free Clinic, the United Way, the Capital Area Agency on Aging, and Richmond Hill, an ecumenical retreat center whose mission is racial reconciliation in the city. Recent publications include *Soulful Aging: Ministry Through the Stages of Adulthood* (with Jane Wilson), and *Thriving Beyond Midlife* (with E. Craig MacBean). He is currently working on the book *Ecology and the Practice of Hope*. Dr. Simmons is the editor of *Religion, Aging, and Spirituality*, a 3,000+ item online annotated bibliography.

CONTENTS

Acknowledgments

This book would not be possible without the participation of hundreds of older adults who provided information about their experiences through interviews, surveys, and formal and informal conversations. They included strangers, friends, and family members. Their sharing of experiences provides the bedrock upon which this framework is based and a view of older adulthood "from the inside." We appreciate the insightful reading of parts of the manuscript by Mernathan Sykes and her efforts to sensitize the authors to the breadth of the older adult experience.

* * *

"I Go On" text by Stephen Schwartz and Leonard Bernstein from *Mass: A Theatre Piece for Singers, Players and Dancers* by Leonard Bernstein. © Copyright 1971 by the Estate of Leonard Bernstein and Stephen Schwartz. Reprinted by permission of Leonard Bernstein Music Publishing Co., LLC, Boosey & Hawkes, Inc., sole licensor.

Introduction

Even those personally and professionally close to persons in the latter part of the journey of life have difficulty entering into a world that is experientially so very distant. They may observe important changes—gradual slowing of metabolism and reaction time, shifts in energy and attitudes, short-term and long-term goals that become more difficult to distinguish, visual physical changes, or diminishing support networks. They may recognize specific events that make this time different from other times of life for a given individual. Particular health challenges, opportunities for extended leisure time, concerns voiced by family members, a death that recasts a person's life—these are some ways in which the latter years of an individual may come to the attention of the helping professional.

But while all these may be realities in the latter years of life, they are unlikely to have the same resonances for the person experiencing them as for the person observing them. The person whose experience it is sees these in a life context that is not primarily framed by the kinds of specific events that bring them to the attention of the helping professional. They may experience more urgency, joy, or anxiety because of a recognition of the reality of death. They may want to make the best of these years in every way, without being quite sure what that entails. They may be puzzled at the lack of clarity about what to expect, as they see some friends who appear to forge ahead into their nineties with great physical and intellectual vigor, and others who appear to slide into a steady physical and psychological decline.

It is critical that the professional understand the world of the older adult from the *inside* as well as from the vantage point of the observer. As the population of older persons continues its dramatic rise, the increasing diversity of the older population in age, culture, interests, health, and other demographic characteristics will present increasing

A Journey Called Aging: Challenges and Opportunities in Older Adulthood
© 2007 by The Haworth Press, Taylor & Francis Group. All rights reserved.
doi:10.1300/5915_01

challenges to perceptions of older adulthood that are strongly influenced by the perspectives of the observer's culture and class. The dilemmas and opportunities to be addressed during the latter years will impact the practice of all who count older persons among their clients, formally or informally, and all who are greatly concerned about a particular older person. These challenges and the choices they engender are increasingly the subject of conversations between older adults and those professionals and others upon whom they rely for assistance and advice.

AUDIENCE

A great many are called upon to assist in the journey through older adulthood. Professionals in health care, medicine, and social work, as well as therapists, psychologists, counselors, educators, ministers, attorneys, financial advisors, program directors, activity coordinators, and facility managers are likely to provide professional services to older adults. In addition, persons with aging relatives, those linked to older persons through extended families or kinship networks, and a host of others may have high involvement with older adults and significant responsibility for their well-being. Most of these, however, lack formal training in gerontology and knowledge of the life changes that older adults may anticipate and experience. As the older segment of the population increases in number and proportion to the whole, the need for professionals to understand the dynamics and sequences of older adulthood will also increase. A recent statement by the American Psychological Association (2004) notes the lack of training of many who serve an older population and underlines the importance of preparation to understand the issues confronted by older adults.

Even those who have tried to prepare themselves to work with older adults may find a gap between the literature and the reality. Much of the professional literature treats older adulthood as if it were a single stage, notwithstanding the possibility that it could encompass as much as a quarter or even a third of a person's years. Often the literature focuses on a moment of crisis, such as a sudden change in well-being, the loss of a spouse, or the need for care, without considering the larger context within which this moment occurs, and its sequence in the overall scheme of events. Professionals may be called upon to provide counsel in decision making or planning without having a clear view themselves of the options that the future may provide.

This book presents an overview of the years between the entry into older adulthood and death and describes a developing context for understanding individual older persons. Despite images of older adulthood that tend to regard all those between the ages of 60 and 90 as a single subpopulation, older persons experience significant changes that distinguish members of this larger age group from one another.

As the journey through the last third of life unfolds, major landmarks appear, present significant challenges, require decisions, and result in a course of action. These landmarks are captured in a framework that begins with entering older adulthood and ends in dying. This framework depicts and interprets three discrete stable periods and two major transitions in older adulthood. Choices and decisions are organized under four large task areas that persist across the journey: to maintain and discover purpose; to hold and build relationships; to balance autonomy, dependence, and interdependence; and to face loss and address change.

This new way of looking at the last third of life brings the professional and other interested persons to an awareness and understanding of the tasks and choices confronting older adults at various stages in their latter years and of the sequence in which they are likely to occur. Building on this awareness, those linked to members of the older adult population increase their capability to be of assistance to those who depend on them in a time of change and challenge.

INDIVIDUAL EXPERIENCE OF AGE

Within the broader outline of this framework and within the four task areas, occurrences specific to each individual can yield a very different experience and outcome during this period of life. The way in which particular individuals age and the choices which they make depend upon a number of factors, some specific to the individuals and others specific to their environment. All of these factors are experienced simultaneously, so that to distinguish the discrete effects of gender, culture, class, or historical context on an individual may be very difficult.

Genetic Makeup

All persons bring their own genetic makeup to the older adult experience. This means that genetically encoded predispositions will impact both an individual's longevity and the way in which that person responds to illness and disease. For example, two people who have diabetes may in late life each come to a dramatically different health status depending in part on their genetic backgrounds. Beyond this, there are also late-life genes that can influence the way people age. Anecdotally, we hear this of families: "That's the way all the Smith women age." Particular strengths in cognition and sharpness of memory may be the result of use as well as genetic heritage.

Gender

Gender also plays a role in how one experiences this time of life. Women tend to live longer than men, on average by seven years, although early indicators suggest that this gap may be narrowing. This means that most women will experience life as a single person. Although women are more likely to replace friendships that are lost in the later years than are men, they will face rigorous challenges alone. Increased longevity, divorce, and widowhood combine to steadily increase the number of single women in this country. Economic realities explain much about the way women experience this time of life differently from men. Women on average have spent less time in the workplace and were paid 30 percent less than their male counterparts. In addition, the death of a husband may mean the loss of economic well-being and social identity as well as the loss of companionship for many women. They therefore may expect different financial outcomes, confirming in many cases the saying that "old women are poor women." In the future, the consequences of a heightened consciousness among women, the recognition of cultural influences in shaping perceptions of women's roles, dramatic advancements in the workplace, and changes in their social roles portend even broader diversity in their lives as older persons.

Culture

Choices that persons make are framed by the cultural traditions from which they come and in which they live. In particular, the beliefs, roles, and values of national, ethnic, or minority groups are important determinants in establishing expectations and shaping the behaviors of group members about growing old and meeting the physical and emotional changes associated with aging. These expectations may also delineate the status and role of an older person. For example, they may specify such responsibilities for older adults as caring for grandchildren and preserving the group's traditions and values by teaching them, plus they may also include the responsibilities of adult children to care for their aging parents. Cultural values and expectations impact, to a greater or lesser degree, a person's adaptation to older adulthood. These same identifying traditions may have been responsible for the marginalization of group members during their youth and adult years.

Cultural values are often reflected in extended family networks or, conversely, in strict lineal family hierarchies, as these kinship organizations participate in members' responses to the changes of older adulthood and as they are impacted by those changes. High rates of immigration from cultures that prize extended family relationships have resulted in a greater level of diversity among the organization and membership of kinship networks.

Since no two ethnic groups are exactly alike in their cultural practices, and since the practices receive varying degrees of adherence by individual members of groups, it is impossible to generalize across the cultural traditions of ethnic minorities. Cultural practices are also impacted by generational differences, by the degree to which individual members of minority groups are assimilated into other and possibly more dominant cultures, and by the historical context in which a group member has lived. Cultural practices differ among similar ethnic groups by geography and by the cohort of group members.

The danger of stereotyping occurs when inferences about individual choices are projected to the larger group. "Culture" is an elusive category, and any attempt to speak for an entire subpopulation has distinct limits. Although one cannot assume the existence of any single dominant culture, common strands and similarities are frequently attributed to a dominant cultural group and are mistakenly regarded as representing a cultural norm. Sensitivity to cultural uniqueness varies among persons and groups; however, consciousness of the distinctiveness of cultural traditions seems to be greater among members of identifiable ethnic and minority groups, and lesser among members of the dominant cultural traditions (Tisdell, 2003, p. 45). Since the older adult population is growing more rapidly among minorities than among whites, behaviors of older adults reflecting distinctive cultural patterns will likely increase as well.

As noted by the National Institute on Aging and the U.S. Census Bureau, the face of aging in the United States will change dramatically in the relatively near future: in numbers, in percentage of the population, in longevity and health, in economic circumstances, in geographic distribution, in social profile, and in diversity by race and Hispanic origin. The implications of these shifts relate to the social and economic impact of the aging of the baby boom generation, changing marital and family makeup, the better education of future cohorts, the fact that women will more likely have their own retirement income as a result of longer tenure in the workforce, and genetic, biological, and physiological research on aging (He, Sengupta, Velkoff, & DeBarros, 2005, pp. 1-4).

Prior Care of Health

Individuals influence the way they come into late old age by the way they have cared for themselves, their minds, spirits, and bodies, throughout adulthood. Many studies link satisfaction in the later years with a positive response to the challenges of middle age. Evidence of bodily abuse through poor attention to self-care (e.g., use of tobacco, poor food choices, lack of exercise) may also impact the health of one's body in the later years. The continuity between health status, both mental and physical, in adulthood and in older adulthood is strong.

Health status throughout adulthood is strongly linked to economic well-being as well as to racial and ethnic identity. Poor health among adults is more likely to be measured among minorities and is highly correlated with poverty or the absence of health insurance. In some cultural groups, the use of alternative or "folk" medicine resources is common. In addition, persons who have been victimized by discrimination in other areas may also have experienced discrimination in their access to health care services. On the other hand, studies have demonstrated the positive relationship between good health and social support throughout life.

Prior care of health combines with genetic makeup to impact the presence of illness and disease during the latter years. "Old" and "sick" are not the same. In the best of all possible worlds, a person would age without mental or physical pathology. Baltes and Baltes (1990) claim that "the important thing to note is that it is pathological incidents that primarily produce a qualitatively different organism in old age and not aging itself" (p. 8). However, even with the best of medical care, the likelihood of failure of a primary organ system increases with age. But not everyone gets sick, not everyone gets equally sick, not everyone gets sick in the same way, and not everyone gets sick at the same time in life. Many persons in this period of life experience health-related deficits, but the difference between one kind of loss and another (e.g., between Lou Gehrig's disease and congestive heart failure) is significant.

Available Resources

Access to a broad range of resources plays a significant role in the way each person will experience older adulthood. "The more resources a person has, the easier it is to anticipate, confront, and adapt to aging losses" (Baltes & Lang, 1997, p. 433). When people suffer losses in their abilities to manage the demands of their environment (e.g., when they cannot bathe because the sides of the tub are too high to negotiate safely), they are faced with several options: they may choose to relocate to an environment that has facilities designed for persons with disabilities; they may modify their present environment by installing a new tub; they may secure an assistive device, hire a professional caregiver, or engage a family member to ensure safe bathing; or they may simply have to live with the situation as it is, depending on the resources available to support their choice. As losses multiply and become more acute, more resources are needed. These resources may be physical, cognitive, emotional, financial, spiritual, or social, and clearly such resources are not distributed evenly throughout the aging population.

Opportunities for older persons with ample discretionary resources are well-publicized, ranging from costly travel opportunities to high-end continuing care retirement communities. These contrast sharply with the resource-modest or resource-poor worlds of most people in this period. There are, after all, not a few resource-poor persons who have to choose between food and medicine and who lack the resources to support the options they may otherwise choose. To summarize Whitman and Purcell (2005),

> Older Americans are an economically diverse group. In 2004, the median income of individuals age 65 and older was $15,199, but incomes varied widely around this average. Twenty-eight percent of Americans 65 or older had incomes of less than $10,000 in 2004, while 10 percent had incomes of $50,000 or more. . . . Poverty among those age 65 and older has fallen from one-in-three older persons in 1960 to one-in-ten today. While the overall rate of poverty is relatively low, it remains high for women, minorities, the less-educated, and those older than 80.

For 22 percent of the older population, Social Security provides their only source of income (Social Security Administration, 2006).

Members of minority groups are more likely to live below the poverty level than are members of the white population. In many instances, the absence of financial resources increases the need for kin to provide caregiving and other forms of assistance. But there are others anticipating care in a family or extended kinship network who may regard financial resources an irrelevant concern in the face of an abundance of spiritual and relational resources.

Those with resources sufficient to exercise virtually any option they choose may not be required to be so diligent in their planning as those with limited resources. Of course, no amount of financial resources can insulate an individual from the demands on mind, soul, and spirit that the challenges of age impose. Likewise, the relative absence of financial resources will almost certainly exacerbate the difficulties inherent in the road ahead. For example, persons with modest social resources may be advised to develop and maintain a support network, and persons with modest financial resources will need to plan for the most efficient utilization of those resources to provide for their own maintenance in advance of that time when services are required.

Readers in cohorts advancing toward older adulthood may be struck by the extent to which the older adult experience is framed by the availability of resources and to plan their adult years in order to garner the range of assets, financial and other, which they deem sufficient to support them in their latter years.

Social Integration

The quality of relationships is another variable. There are people of very modest means who have the strong support of family or close friends, and who manage well during the periods and changes of older adulthood. Some individuals manage to stay embedded in an extended family or a network of familiar support until the very end of their lives. Others, remarkably, are able to replace lost relationships with new sources of support and engagement. And of course still others never recover from the loss of persons close to them and spend their days in loneliness and isolation. Staying socially integrated is a key to the successful navigation of what may otherwise be difficult times.

How one views social integration in families is conditioned both by cultural expectations and by economic resources. In some cultures, a premium is placed on autonomy and social independence, even in old age. In others, the expectation of support from inclusion in an extended family or surrogate family is paramount. While some older persons expect to be cared for by their children, others insist that they do not want to be a burden to them.

The Setting of Care

How one will experience older adulthood also depends on the time of the onset of frailty and the setting in which care is received. If that setting is a nursing home, there is a vast range in quality of care. A recently launched pilot program of the Center for Medicare and Medicaid Services now has patient care data on the nation's nursing homes available on the Medicare program's Web site, which can be accessed at http://www.Medicare.gov/NHCompare (U.S. Department of Health and Human Services, n.d.). If the context of care is an assisted-living facility, there is also a wide range in quality of services. However, the fact that a person is able to function in assisted living (rather than needing nursing-home care) may already indicate a higher level of functioning in everyday living. If the context of care is one's own residence or that of a member of the family or kinship network, the experience of care is again markedly different from either of the aforementioned environments and may be the result of prior planning or limited resources coupled with a higher level of functioning.

In addition to one's level of functioning, choices surrounding location of care are usually the product of available resources, prior planning, and cultural expectations. In addition, for some, there are issues of access related both to class and to the convenient availability of the services required.

The Geography of Care

How one experiences this time also depends on whether care is received in an urban or a rural setting. A person in a rural area from which there has been substantial out-migration is not in the same situation as the person in an urban setting. Substantial out-migration, low population density, and low median incomes of residents in non-metropolitan areas may combine to cause an absence of institutional resources. Some settings have a wealth of resources—geriatric and gerontological specialists, professionals with skill and experience serving this population, a broad array of institutions sensitive to the unique needs of older persons, social programs designed to provide assistance to those needing it—whereas in other settings a person must travel considerable distance to obtain these services. Furthermore, older adults, particularly minorities, who live in nonmetropolitan areas are more likely to live in poverty. How one experiences older adulthood depends in part on the services and resources available and accessible in a particular place.

Cohort

The historical circumstances of youth and adulthood influence each generation of older adults. For some, defining moments have been the Great Depression or World War II. For others, it may have been the confinement of Japanese-American citizens during World War II, or the passage of civil rights legislation, or the controversy surrounding the war in Vietnam. In any case, the circumstances of a particular time and place impact the values and perspectives of those who have lived during a particular historical event or context.

Some cohorts, by virtue of defining events, or by virtue of their size and influence on the entire population, have assumed a unique identity. The World War II cohort, thanks to a recent book tribute to them, has been dubbed "the greatest generation." The earliest of those born in the late 1940s, 1950s, and early 1960s, known as the "baby boom generation," are just entering older adulthood, and as more of the 77 million persons in this cohort follow, they will likely place their own stamp on this time of life, given their past record of creating lifestyle, social, and cultural change.

Developmental and Other Disabilities

The presence of any of a broad range of cognitive, physical, or emotional impairments may not necessarily shorten one's life expectancy, but it certainly frames both the options available to an older person and that person's ability to make choices. It also increases the likelihood that significant care will be required. Depending on the nature and severity of the disability, opportunities related to meaning, relationships, and autonomy and dependency may take a unique shape or be all but impossible to consider.

Sexual Orientation

Although same-sex and opposite-sex older couples share many of the same characteristics, those participating in lesbian, gay, bisexual, and transgender relationships commonly face particular problems in older adulthood resulting from discrimination, social and health services unresponsive to alternative lifestyles, and obligations in a partnership that may not be legally recognized (Berger & Kelly, 2000, p. 62).

This vast array of areas describing potential individual differences may lead the reader to the conclusion that no framework can possibly capture the diversity of experience comprised by older adulthood. However, just the opposite is the case. The breadth and source of individual differences prompt such a study in order to identify the commonalities contained within that experience. Individual differences notwithstanding, by using this book as a guide, the reader will gain a comprehensive view of this part of the life span set within an orderly framework and thereby can recognize the challenges and choices that occur to individuals during the older adult years. This book emphasizes both common patterns as well as the individual differences derived from gender, socioeconomic status, culture, and context. But between the common patterns and individual differences, there is a vast fertile area, filled with challenges, yet presenting the occasions to make these years rich and rewarding.

OVERVIEW

Instead of viewing this as a time of continuous decline, consider it a time of relative stability, punctuated by major challenges and changes. *A Journey Called Aging* is organized to present these changes in the order in which they are likely to occur. Chapter 1, "Mapping the Journey," presents the research upon which the book is based. Chapter 2, "Entering Older Adulthood," begins the sequence by describing the events which begin the journey through older adulthood. Chapter 3, "Extended Middle Age," describes the first stable period. Chapter 4, "The Early Transition," introduces the dramatic changes that interrupt the flow of the first stable period by forcing reorganization and the setting of new priorities. Chapter 5, "An Older Adult Lifestyle," describes a revised lifestyle in which people identify themselves with others who are in this period and adapt themselves to it. Chapter 6, "The Later Transition," describes the transposition from autonomy to increased dependency and/or interdependency. Chapter 7, "While the Light Lasts," describes the stable time near the end of life, and Chapter 8, "Dying Well," describes the final transition, death. The epilogue presents a challenge to all to encourage and assist older persons to prevail over the vicissitudes of the latter years as persons of compassion and sacrifice and endurance.

Chapter 1

Mapping the Journey

Would anyone choose to be old? Would any 40-year-old elect to be 60, or any 60-year-old want to be 80? Occasionally working adults envy the perceived leisure time of retirees, but in contemporary culture age is usually coveted only when compared to the alternative. Instead of being sought, aging is usually viewed as a time thrust upon an individual as if it were either a burden or a gift of dubious value.

In the popular imagination, aging begins in the fifties or sixties, usually after full-time employment of oneself and/or one's spouse, and comprises the final major segment of one's life. For a good many, this time amounts to the last quarter of life; for an increasing number, it is the last third. For some, it is a time of eager anticipation, filled with the promise of opportunities contained in life's capstone; for others, it is a time of resignation, if not dread, that whatever promise life holds has passed.

Some people respond to the thought of their own older years by planning for this stage of life, no matter how welcome or unwelcome, just as they might plan for any other time. Some pretend that middle age will continue ad infinitum and that the difficult changes the older years portend will not happen to them. Others cloak themselves within traditions of family or culture that have historically prescribed life in older adulthood and that for them continue to do so.

The professional who serves older persons is faced with individuals in many different contexts: the person who has made plans, the person who refuses to plan, and the person who feels no need to plan. While it is beyond the capacity of this book and the research upon which it is based to address all of the situations reflected in this diversity, it can

A Journey Called Aging: Challenges and Opportunities in Older Adulthood
© 2007 by The Haworth Press, Taylor & Francis Group. All rights reserved.
doi:10.1300/5915_02

nevertheless provide a framework for the professional to anticipate and understand the events and the needs that persons experience during their older adult years.

LANDMARKS ON THE ROAD AHEAD

Each phase of life—childhood, adolescence, adulthood, and older adulthood—has its own rhythm. Most theorists agree that frameworks exist that help us understand the constants, the complexities, and the changes that occur. These changes may be considered developmental in the sense that earlier events and changes help shape subsequent ones. Their significance is derived from the interaction between an individual and various elements of the environment, both internal and external. Furthermore, the meaning of events and changes is largely in the eye of the beholder, making their interpretation a key element of their significance.

Hultsch and Deutsch (1981) note that the developmental process of aging

> may be viewed as a series of transitions defined by . . . events [with] different events . . . important to different people. Each event is like a snapshot which conveys some of the raw meaning of adult life. But in another sense, these snapshots are isolated personal experiences with little meaning outside of themselves. (p. 7)

Schlossberg (1977) depicts these changes as occurring mainly in the areas of vocation, intimacy, family life, community, and the inner life (p. 79). What gives meaning to the chain of events that marks older adult development is the context in which each occurs, a context informed strongly by traditions of culture and class, and a context in which each individual creates the meaning that surrounds the event. On the one hand, each event may be seen as the raw stuff of which part of life is made, intrinsically little more than a piece of data. At the same time, the events of older adulthood take on the larger meaning that individuals and groups bring to them, tempered by the interplay of gender, color, ethnicity, economic class, location, and lived experiences.

Any framework that describes the older adult years will balance times of transition and times of stability, events that signal change with those that emphasize a steady and continuing pace with strong links to the past and an openness to the future. Such a framework will make space for individual and group differences as well as interpretations of the significance of events. Differences born of gender, ethnicity, culture, and class as well as the heterogeneity that comes from a lifetime of experience may make a single narrow path of older adult development seem impossible. Yet older adults do have experiences in common that, when taken together, serve to describe stability and change in *A Journey Called Aging*. Huyck and Hoyer (1982) judge such conceptual frameworks to be valuable "because they impose some order on what often seem to be chaotic, complex life experiences" (p. 12).

The Cadence of Adulthood

Levinson, Darrow, Klein, Levinson, and McKee (1978) and Levinson and Levinson (1996) have described the cadence of adulthood in terms of transitions or changes that move a person from one period to another. Levinson (1986) theorized that to understand the course of a life, one must "take account of stability and change, continuity and discontinuity, orderly progression as well as stasis and chaotic fluctuation" (p. 3). He and his colleagues (1978) wrote, "A transition is a bridge, or boundary zone, between two states of greater stability. It involves a process of change, a shift from one structure to another" (pp. 49-50). Levinson (1986) characterized the tasks of a transitional or structure-changing period that ordinarily lasts about five years as "to reappraise the existing structure, to explore possibilities for change in the self and the world, and to move toward commitment to the crucial choices that form the basis for a new life structure in the ensuing period" (p. 7). The tasks of a structure-building or stable period are "to form a life structure and enhance our life with it . . . make certain key choices, form a structure around them, and pursue our values and goals within this structure" (p. 7). This structure-building period, though stable, is not necessarily tranquil. Ordinarily it lasts five to seven years, ten at the most, in the period from age 20 to age 60.

Other theorists find greater variance in the timing and duration of transitions and in the degree to which they represent major structural reorganization rather than simply the continuing accumulation of experience (Troll, 1982, p. 7).

But aging is about more than change. Another important element is continuity—what Erik Erikson (1997) called an "invariable core," the "existential identity that is an integration of past, present and future" (p. 9). Continuity provides those links to history and experience that enable both problem solving and meaning. Kaufman (1986) describes it this way:

> Old people formulate and reformulate personal and cultural symbols of their past to create a meaningful, coherent sense of self, and in the process they create a viable present. In this way, the ageless self emerges: its definition is ongoing, continuous, and creative. (p. 14)

The Cadence of Older Adulthood

Likewise, older adulthood has its own rhythm. Perhaps the most popular approach to charting older adult development is the use of chronological age, designating time frames by arbitrarily chosen ages, or in dividing the population on the basis of age into the "young-old" and the "old-old." However, at any discrete chronological age members of the older adult population will reflect a broad heterogeneity. At any chronological age, matters of health, activity, and interest are highly divergent, making chronological age an unreliable predictor of any aspect of the rhythm of the latter years. Most developmental theorists have regarded chronological age as an imprecise measure of most characteristics of older adulthood.

Despite broad awareness of the heterogeneity of the older adult population, most references in the professional literature treat older adulthood as if it were a single life stage, or two at most. Erikson's (1950) eighth stage, "Integrity vs. Despair," is most frequently cited in describing older adulthood. At this stage, a person's task is to resolve the tension between affirming the value of one's years and despairing of their meaninglessness. Interviewed when an octogenarian, Erikson admitted to some surprise at the creative potential and generativity of older adults. He recalled that when he developed his theory, not only was the general image of old age different, but he lacked the capacity to imagine himself becoming old (Hall, 1983). More recently, Joan Erikson (1997) has suggested that increased life expectancy necessitates the reexamination of the stages of the entire life span from the perspective of elders in what she calls the ninth stage (pp. 106-114). Speaking from her own experience, she noted, "Old age in one's eighties and nineties brings with it new demands, reevaluations, and daily difficulties. These concerns can only be adequately discussed, and confronted, by designating a new ninth stage to clarify the challenges" (p. 105). Her addition to her husband's eight stages effectively divides older adulthood into two life stages. Although her discussion of the ninth stage fails to bring forth a new and different task beyond resolving the continuing tension between integrity and despair, Jean Erikson describes as characteristic of this time the loss of capacities, loss of relationship, disintegration, focus on daily functioning, and the need to trust (p. 113).

Havighurst (1952) also describes older adulthood as a single stage, "later maturity," during which older adults are faced with a series of developmental tasks related to spouse, home, family, occupation, community, and social groups.

Peck (1956) amplifies Erikson's eighth stage by dividing it into two periods, each containing a series of tensions to be resolved. Within the first period, "Middle Age," he proposes four tensions to be resolved: "Valuing Wisdom vs. Valuing Physical Powers," "Socializing vs. Sexualizing in Human Relationships," "Cathectic Flexibility vs. Cathectic Impoverishment," and "Mental Flexibility vs. Mental Rigidity." The second period, "Old Age," contained three tensions for resolution: "Ego Differentiation vs. Work-Role Preoccupation," "Body Transcendence vs. Body Preoccupation," and "Ego Transcendence vs. Ego Preoccupation." Peck notes that these psychological tasks and adjustments occur during their respective periods but in different time sequences for different individuals.

Levinson and colleagues (1978) claim that it is "an oversimplification to regard the entire span of years after age 50 or 65 as a single era. Given the lack of research data, we can only speculate about this concluding segment of the life cycle" (p. 38). They therefore suggest dividing older adulthood into two sequential stages: "Late Adulthood," characterized by bodily decline, frequency of death and serious illness among friends, reductions in heavy responsibilities, changed relationships between oneself and society, and living in phase with one's own generation, and "Late, Late Adulthood," where a person's life is marked by infirmity, coming to terms with death, and engaging in an ultimate involvement with oneself. In other words, Levinson and his colleagues speculated, without supporting empirical data, that older adulthood would consist of two stages, the first a time comprising several transitions, and the second, a stable period prior to death. Although older persons were not included among those from whom they gathered data, they (Levinson et al., 1978) expected that the alternating sequence of transition and stability would continue among older adults in the two periods he called "Late Adulthood" and "Late, Late Adulthood." This two-stage approach of Levinson and his colleagues plus the one suggested earlier by Joan Erikson as a ninth stage reflect some awareness of both the length and heterogeneity of the older adult experience.

The challenges professionals face in their work with this segment of the population are exacerbated by the absence of research-based signposts to identify stages in the rhythm of the latter years. Experience provides ample evidence that a person 65 years of age and a person 85 years of age are at different places in the scheme of older adulthood, with differences in their experiences and capabilities. Despite commonalities, they will also possess divergent perspectives on their location on the path between middle adulthood and death. The identification of markers to guide one through periods of stability and times of change provided the impetus for the research upon which this work is based.

THE RESEARCH

In the empirical study that serves as the foundation for this book, Fisher (1993) examined the lives of 74 older adults, aged 61 to 94, using interview data that described the events that had occurred to them and the context in which these events derived meaning. The initial purpose of the research was to examine life stories and to probe the significance of experiences and the context in which significance occurred for those telling the stories. The interviews occurred at two senior centers, an adult learning center, and eight private residences in an urban county, and at two senior centers and a nursing home located in adjacent counties comprising rural and suburban communities; 70 percent of those interviewed were female; the mean age of the sample was 78; 5 percent of those interviewed were African American. The mean level of educational attainment was twelfth grade, and 78 percent had been employed in nonprofessional occupations prior to retirement.

This sample is consistent with the total national population of older adults in several important respects: it is predominately female, and the average level of educational attainment is twelfth grade. Furthermore, the mean age of the sample approximates the average life expectancy of the American population.

Data from the interviews were coded to identify pivotal events, common themes, clusters of experience, and significant changes described by the participants. As story after story unfolded, transitions that disrupted, redirected, or dramatically changed an individual's life flow emerged and grounded a framework upon which other events were located. The first of these transitions came somewhat early in older adulthood. It was usually triggered by a serious illness, the death of a spouse, or the need to relocate—all events that brought new priorities to the fore. "After my husband died . . ." or "When he took sick . . ." became hinge expressions introducing both discontinuity and redirection. In instances where individuals and married couples introduced change into their lives voluntarily, the events of the transition served as catalysts to alter the tempo, the organization, and the focus of life and, in some instances, the location. The second transition came somewhat later in older adulthood. It was marked by phrases such as "When I was no longer able to care for myself . . ." that signified an abrupt change both in lifestyle and location. This transition marks the inability of an individual to maintain autonomy and the need for increased dependence on others for various levels of assistance.

Periods of adjustment to new goals and priorities and ensuing stability occurred after each of these transitions. Participants in the study reported a stable period of extended middle age prior to the first transition. Between the first and second transitions, there occurred a period of stability in which persons established themselves as older adults. The second transition was followed by a final stable period in which persons established themselves as dependent older adults. Entry into the time described by these five periods usually occurs with retirement or by dint of age, and exit occurs with death. No data were gathered to gauge the length of either transitional or stable periods.

The following is the sequence of the five periods:

1. *Extended Middle Age*
   • Middle age lifestyle continued
   • Goals for retirement pursued
   • Other activities substituted for or combined with work
2. *Early Transition*
   • Involuntary transitional events
   • Voluntary transitional events
   • End of continuity with middle age
3. *Older Adult Lifestyle*
   • Adaptation to changes of early transition
   • Stable lifestyle consistent with older adult status
   • Socialization realized through age group affiliation
4. *Later Transition*
   • Loss of autonomy
   • Loss of health and mobility
   • Need for assistance and/or care
5. *Final Period*
   • Adaptation to changes of later transition
   • Stable lifestyle appropriate to level of dependency
   • Sense of finitude, mortality

The flow of transition interrupting stability also brings about a sequence of endings, often occurring with the loss of the familiar, and beginnings that contain the prospect of growth and renewal. This flow in and of itself has the immense capacity to transform a life, as certain circumstances and roles are discontinued and new ones are born. It serves to eliminate some of the unnecessary baggage carried from earlier days, lifting the weight of priorities set in earlier periods that have since become burdens. The notion that these periods may be anticipated, even charted in the latter years, provides professionals and others with a backdrop against which to view the needs and decisions faced by older adult clients, friends, and family members.

A Descriptive Framework

Discussions of developmental patterns, particularly among adults and older adults, inevitably raise questions concerning the descriptive versus the prescriptive nature of the pattern. Did the life events of every participant in the research study fit the framework completely? No. Is the one who does not fit abnormal? No. But the framework does describe the experience of most participants in the study together with their spouses. As such its value is in being descriptive and instructive.

There were three major exceptions to completing the framework among those involved in the study. The most common exception occurred among spouses of participants who failed to live long enough to complete all of the periods of the framework. Since a majority of the study participants were widows/widowers, they were able to recount the life stories of spouses who had died during one of the intervening periods.

A second exception occurred among persons who "fast-forwarded" through the periods, in particular moving from a period of autonomy to a period of dependency early in older adulthood. A person who was seriously injured late in adulthood and no longer able to care for himself or herself entered the Later Transition without first experiencing Extended Middle Age, the Early Transition, or the Older Adult Lifestyle.

A third exception occurred among a few widows and widowers who, having experienced the death of a spouse during the Early Transition, remarried and reverted to the period of Extended Middle Age. This was, of course, a temporary exception, since they would confront the Early Transition and subsequent periods once again at some point in their lives together as a married couple, and then they would continue through subsequent periods, assuming they lived that long.

Another kind of temporary exception occurs when persons in the early periods are temporarily incapacitated or handicapped, temporarily by virtue of injury or accident, placing them briefly in the Later Transition, but who upon recovery reverted to their former period.

However, even when the developmental paths of particular individuals are not in complete conformity with the sequence of the framework, the events and tasks linked to the periods of the framework are nevertheless likely to be confronted during older adulthood, assuming an individual lives long enough.

The content of *A Journey Called Aging* combines a developmental sequence with the events and tasks of the various periods. As a result, the benefit of this book to the reader, whether a professional or one interested in learning about this time of life, may be for some to suggest a framework for planning the sequence of the latter years, or it may be for others to call attention to those tasks and events that are likely to be confronted in every older adult experience.

Rationale

The increase in numbers of older persons together with improvements in their well-being and advances in their longevity during the past half century has served to focus attention on older adulthood. However, interest in successful aging has not been matched by curiosity about the developmental sequences occurring in older adulthood. One may view human development much as a fifteenth-century medieval map of the world where some parts are carefully detailed (child and adult youth development, for example), but other parts (such as the older years) are only partially and vaguely mapped at best, or are simply identified as terra incognita. The framework derived from this study provides a useful starting point for further investigation into the developmental sequences experienced by an aging population.

As individuals venture into this uncharted territory, they bring concerns about living within their means and maintaining their health. They also bring fears of change, losing autonomy, and suffering. But more important, they bring the need for worthwhile and meaningful activity, interesting experiences, and supportive companions. For some, the older adult experience is viewed from an individual perspective, as though it occurred mainly to a person or to a partnership; for others, the older adult experience is seen as a group experience, occurring within the context of a lineal or extended family network, in which changes impact both the individual and the kinship relationships and structure.

A Journey Called Aging presents a framework within which to organize plans and base expectations so that the promise within the gift of years may be realized for each older person. It may serve as a guide for professionals and others who care for or about older persons, examining periods that bring change as well as periods that are settling. It may help to create a balanced outlook suggesting priorities beyond busyness or relaxation, thereby aiding in developing a perspective, shaping a vision, and designing a plan for the enrichment of the journey to life's end. It may also highlight the crucial role that preparation of every sort plays in the quality of life on the road ahead, as well as the almost inevitable burdens that scarcity of resources will impose.

For the professional who interacts with older adults and all those who care about them, this book can be both a teaching tool and interpretative framework, helping to make sense of the changes that older adults go through, and suggesting options to help all concerned move past the merely physical to the fully human, where loss and death are recognized and where freedom, choices, meaning, and relationships continue to be core parts of the journey of life.

THE TASKS ON THE ROAD AHEAD

Our focus shifts now from the structure of the latter years, expressed as times of transition and times of stability, to the dynamics of the latter years, captured in tasks that make up the agenda and are the stuff of which life in this time is made. *A Journey Called Aging* gathers these tasks into four large task areas: discovering purpose, building and maintaining relationships, balancing autonomy with dependence and interdependence, and facing loss and addressing change.

Like the structure, the tasks are descriptive, not prescriptive. They are pervasive without fitting each person like a glove and describe in broad strokes the needs, challenges, and preoccupations of older persons, as well as the opportunities. In a sense, they capture the continuing business of living. For example, few persons could be described as being completely devoid of purpose and relationships; yet questions such as "Who am I, now that I am 70 or 80 or 90 years old?" and "Why am I still here?" permeate conversations as well as interviews. Loneliness resulting from the absence of good relationships tops many lists of older adult concerns. Living with the right proportions of independence and dependence as one grows older and likely more frail, and dealing with significant changes and losses, both those experienced and those anticipated, are paramount concerns. The precise shape of each of these task areas as well as their respective levels of importance to an individual depend on individual factors such as life experiences, gender, culture, and class, as well as on the particular period in the framework in which the person is living. Each task is modified by each transition and stable period.

Consequently, in these broadly outlined task areas are found the threads woven throughout older adulthood, appearing and reappearing, emerging from the experiences of persons living in these years. Joan Erikson (1997) reminds us that the tasks and tensions that are initially consigned to earlier life stages nevertheless reappear to individuals in their latter years (p. 106).

Professionals and family members often become aware of the aging process of another as they become involved directly with one of these tasks. Rarely, of course, does the task area appear with such a neat label as "purpose" or "autonomy." In fact, these abstractions are likely never used. But what does occur is a conversation in which a person mourns recent retirement because retirement "is even more boring than work." Or a family meets to discuss what to do with Mother, who insists on living alone in the family home, although members of the family agree that it is dangerous for her to continue to do so. The tasks emerge not as discrete topics for discussions in a "seminar on older adulthood," but they appear in the forms of major crises, daily decisions, and greater or lesser concerns with which older persons wrestle and around which family members, older persons, and professionals interact.

It is the purpose of *A Journey Called Aging* to make the task areas recognizable by discussing their dynamic and describing experiences as they have occurred to older persons in different situations and in different periods of older adulthood. What is of particular import is the way in which each task area changes across the changes and transitions of these years. Relationships, for example, are different when a person is in good health and socially active than when that person is bedridden and provided for in an extended-care facility. Issues surrounding autonomy and dependence take on a new urgency when a person is no longer able to live alone, or in a cultural tradition where interdependence is valued more greatly than autonomy.

In addition to interviews conducted in more formal research set- tings, scores of people have shared stories about their experience as older adults. Those stories, gathered over decades of attentive listening, are shared in *A Journey Called Aging* to give flesh to these task areas and to illumine experiences of concern and interest to older adults, family members, and professionals.

The framework upon which the book is based divides the lengthy stage of older adulthood into five periods. These periods are book-ended at the beginning with the entry into older adulthood, often through retirement, and at the end by death. Between retirement and death, an older person may experience five different periods reflecting sequences in the older adult experience. The tasks recur in each of those periods, taking different shapes and providing different levels of concern or challenge for different individuals. A brief overview of these four task areas is introduced in the following pages.

To Balance Autonomy with Dependence

The perspective from which one views this group of tasks is molded to a large degree by the combined influences of culture and class. In no other task area do these influences play such a significant role. Those with ample resources generally regard autonomy as a value; they experience it mainly as individuals or in a partnership and guard it until that time when they can no longer maintain themselves and must depend on others. Where autonomy is prized, retirement communities, cohousing, extended care facilities, nursing homes, home care assistants, and others are likely to be engaged to provide services to older persons, preserving some level of independence and thereby allowing them "not to be a burden" to their children or families for care. Others, especially members of minority groups and those with limited resources, tend to experience interdependence as a lifelong member of an extended family, where complete independence occurs only when one exits that family relationship, and where the mutual sharing of limited resources through a network of linear, consanguineous, and fictive ties binds groups of persons together. Where interdependence is the chief value, the extended family is expected to care for an individual in the latter years just as it has provided a caring network that included that individual throughout youth and adulthood. Among some cultural groups, reliance upon institutions as caregivers may serve to stigmatize an extended family as unable or unwilling to care for its own. While different groups of older persons may be identified as adhering to each of these as juxtaposed values, a great many also value both of them: some level of autonomy is sought in order to retain a measure of control over one's choices, and at the same time, some level of support or caregiving is expected to be provided by an immediate or extended family.

This discussion of task areas begins with autonomy, not because it is more important than the others, but because the assumption that persons have choices is fundamental to the premise of this book. It is also an issue underlying many of the concerns about which professionals interact with older persons. Professionals and others often experience the temperament of these years on the sharp edge of claims of autonomy. Disagreements over choices of action often focus on who owns a particular decision or who will decide how one should cope with changes or losses. Planning for the stages of older adulthood assumes that individuals have the independence and the support necessary to make and implement their plans, recognizing that the plans cover periods that involve increasing levels of dependency.

What influences might frame such choices? The societal web of what it means to be an older adult may present obstacles. Stereotyped messages of the media about what older persons need (usually medical and personal care products), how older persons behave (passively and at a reduced pace), and what older adults expect (a discount) can impose a perspective that dampens if not reduces options. Cultural values of a particular ethnic group as articulated by family members or friends may serve to prescribe the roles available to older persons. As a result, issues related to choices often wend their way through the complicated maze of family and group relationships and traditions. Some cultural traditions value independence on the part of older persons: "The last thing I want is to be a burden to my children." Others value the opposite: "The last thing I want is for Mother to be in a nursing home; we will care for her in our home until she dies." Clearly the availability of resources establishes parameters around the choices that an individual may make. Furthermore, as Carol Gilligan (1982) points out, women in particular may experience a conflict between autonomy and compassion, "denying responsibility by claiming only to meet the needs of others," while struggling "to reclaim the self and to solve the moral problem in such a way that no one is hurt" (p. 71).

If autonomy in older adulthood represents one end of a continuum, dependency represents the other. To be dependent is to rely on others for support or care, ranging from talking with friends and family prior to making an important decision to living in a nursing home where all of one's needs are met. Neither autonomy nor dependence are absolutes, nor is there an optimal or prescribed point between them designed to ensure successful aging. However, as Krout and Pillemer (2003) observe,

> Negotiating the ambivalence between increasing needs for help and support from others on the one hand and the desire to remain independent and in control of one's life on the other is one of the key dynamics of the aging process. It is in its potential to alleviate the dilemma between dependence and autonomy that supportive living arrangements play such a critical role. (p. 198)

Health status, cultural expectations, a supportive environment, and availability of resources all impact a person's place on this continuum between autonomy and dependence.

A distortion of the balance between autonomy and dependence occurs in the widespread belief by some that this is a time of relief from decision making. For some, it may mean that there is only the need to make appropriate pension and/or Social Security options, update one's will, and then coast—responding and reacting to whatever opportunities and calamities each day presents. For others, it may be the time to surround oneself with a loving and caring family and depend entirely on them to make whatever decisions are necessary. One gentleman, reflecting on his stay in a nursing home, said, "Here, they make all of your decisions for you." And for those with limited financial resources who are convinced that they have no alternatives, there is the challenge of identifying choices that they can afford to implement.

With the passing of full-time employment and parenting, life is often described as freedom from responsibilities, freedom from early rising, freedom from a fixed schedule, freedom from caring for children, and so on. But this view is one-sided at best: it includes only what is left behind, and not what stands ahead. Freedom *from* is, in itself, inadequate.

Autonomy as a cultural value bespeaks a certain degree of individualism. It is about deciding for oneself, making choices, setting direction, and speaking one's voice. It refers to the courage to be true to oneself, to be unfettered and forthright, to uncover family secrets and address social ills, and to claim one's own fragile truth. For some, it refers to the ability to develop a script or a lifestyle that satisfies their needs. Autonomy is about the attitude and stance one takes vis-à-vis the constraints—real or untested—that would limit one's field of options. The ability to make personal as well as ethical choices depends on it. As such, it comprises a range of attitudes, postures, and decisions that determine the size of a person's universe, the degree of self-reliance and self-esteem upon which commitments are based, and the degree to which persons can shape their lives.

One 76-year-old reflected:

> When I was in my mid-sixties, I started to venture forth with my observations and raise questions few people were asking. By that time, it didn't matter to me whether others agreed with me, only that I speak the truth as I saw it. At long last, I knew I had something to say—or rather, I knew there were things that needed to be said and I had to join the few who were saying them. (Lustbader, 2001, p. 216)

Autonomy reflects a freedom *for* that completes the equation by describing the challenges faced and choices made in the quest for fulfillment. Peter, now caregiver for his wife, surprises himself with his willingness and ability to do hands-on care: "I didn't know I had it in me." Clyde and Angie, retired teachers, relocated to a small town without a bookstore. With no business experience to speak of, they decided to put their time and resources into a brand-new venture: opening a bookstore to serve their area. Sophie Ann, nursing-home resident for 18 months, has just discovered a love for and talent at writing stories: "I've got something to say and I'm going to say it before I die." Miki, whose first language is Korean, decided to develop her English language proficiency, although her children asked her, "Why does an old woman like you need to go back to school? Stay home and care for the children." And Pearl is working at the child care center, knowing that her daughter and son-in-law can't afford to support an extra person in their home without her income. These people are wrestling with opportunities born in autonomy, with choosing who to be, with speaking their own voices, with deciding how to live amid dramatically new and changing circumstances, with choosing. One senses various levels of autonomy as these persons make choices regarding their older adult vocations. The challenge of enjoying autonomy and expressing greater personal mastery occurs within each of the periods of the framework, as over time persons become increasingly dependent upon others and upon their environment.

To Discover Purpose

The move from the productivity of middle age adulthood to the purpose of older adulthood is a shift from answers to questions. One of the great challenges of the older adult years is to find one's place, one's niche, one's role, one's voice. An inner commitment to freedom provides the environment both to search for and decide upon such a place. Joseph Campbell (1988) claimed that

[p]eople say that what we're all seeking is a meaning for life. I don't think that's what we're really seeking. I think that what we're seeking is an experience of being alive, so that our life experiences on the purely physical plane will have resonances within our own innermost being and reality so that we actually feel the rapture of being alive. (p. 5)

As the quest for life endures throughout these years, even to their end, to be alive and to have a purpose for being alive make the years an awesome gift.

Harry R. Moody (1986) suggests that there are "three distinct strands woven into the search for the meaning of life at the level of individual autobiography . . . that my life be understandable, that it be purposeful, and that it be happy" (p. 26). At the individual level, Moody's conditions make this task practical and manageable, pointing the older adult to such basics as the what, the why, and the how of living.

Nearly all enter older adulthood with some sense of meaning and purpose, with years filled with experiences aimed at making their lives understandable, purposeful, and happy. And if there are outside forces to be engaged in this quest for meaning, drawn from religion, philosophy, or nature, then it is likely that older persons are acquainted with these sources as well. As a result, any discussion of meaning or purpose occurs against the backdrop of a lifetime of experience.

Nevertheless, searching for meaning is one of those deep human strivings that persist, and any sense of purpose is challenged by each of the changes and challenges that older adulthood brings.

> Marjory was the vice president of finance for a small manufacturing firm. She loved numbers and detailed facts. After her retirement, she kept up with the financial news each day and with friends she had known in the business community. But over time, her friends passed away, and her vision was stolen by macular degeneration. An avid lifetime reader, she refuses to listen to books on tape. In her darkness, she lives alone in a small apartment in a care facility, calling her children frequently because she has nothing else to do.

Contrast Marjory with Shona:

> Shona lives with her daughter, her granddaughter, a niece, and two great-grandchildren. From time to time her brother stops by for a few days in the crowded apartment. Since all of the adults in this extended family have work responsibilities except Shona, it is expected that she will provide child care for the two little ones, as well as for the children of other family members nearby. Shona is able to remember how her great-grandmother cared for her when she was that age. For a 70-year-old, caring for two and sometimes three or four children fills all of her time. There is no time to ponder purpose—it is a given—in her extended family.

The question of meaning may take shape, for example, in a very practical inner dialogue: What am I to do, now that I no longer have family and work to occupy me? What am I to do, now that my circumstance has changed? Isn't this my time—time I've earned for myself to do whatever I want? Yes, but isn't this my last chance to make a difference? What are older people supposed to be doing? These questions may recur with each transition and stable period, and the answers may or may not be a given.

How these questions are answered speaks to purpose, whether purpose for that individual is envisioned as enrichment, service, entertainment, achievement, adventure, or contemplation. Discovery for some is the key word: discovering purpose, determining order, considering the alternatives. For others, it is adoption: adopting the purpose that one's parents and grandparents and all of the other older people in one's extended family or community have assumed.

Cultural expectations informing one's sense of autonomy will likely point in one of these directions. The time calls for purpose, however long or short the years remaining. For some, the process flows as distractions lessen. Looking back, one person put it this way:

> When you're young, you've got too much going on. There's no way to comprehend it all. Everything is coming at you at once. Life is a blur. . . . Gradually things settle down. You're less distracted. You're finally able to decide where to focus your attention. You start to pin things down and take a good look at them. That's where you can really see what's going on. (Lustbader, 2001, p. 224)

Purpose is also developed from participation in particular communities of meaning: religious, social, recreational, and volunteer groups all serve to provide reasons for living. What persons believe, what they value, and purpose are all products of the families in which they have lived, the ethnic and cultural groups of which they are part, their gender, the way of life they and their friends enjoy, and the time during which they have lived. Life meanings are not the possession of individuals: they have about them a "held in common" dimension arising from the groups and cultures from which they have emerged and in which they still hold membership.

Simone de Beauvoir (1972) in *The Coming of Age* contends that

> [t]here is only one solution if old age is not to be an absurd parody of our former life, and that is to go on pursuing ends that give our existence a meaning—devotion to individuals, to groups or to causes, social, political, intellectual or creative work. (p. 540)

Discovery, affirmation, adoption—by whatever key words—questions of meaning and affirmations of purpose lead and pursue through the periods of older adulthood. As with the other task areas, this one is also reshaped in each transition and in each stable period. In every period, having goals and moving to achieve them contribute to the happiness and satisfaction of older persons. And while few professionals or family members will be engaged in a discussion about a topic as abstract as "the meaning of life," they will be caught up in situations where older people are bored or depressed because they have nothing interesting to do, because they are "sick and tired of looking at the same four walls day after day." After an adulthood of busyness with career, family, or just keeping the body and soul together, where purpose was so integral to living that it may never have been consciously chosen, being relieved of those responsibilities may introduce a vacuum in which reasons for living must be rediscovered or adopted anew.

To Build Relationships

People need other people for both a sense of well-being and a sense of identity. Close emotional ties with a network of family members and friends is an essential component of a sense of well-being and contentment. Intimacy is a critical part of human happiness, whether that is spousal intimacy, the closeness of friends, or the social support of adult children and members of an extended family. One gentleman expressed his good fortune this way: "My wife is my best friend and lifelong companion. Every time I look at her, I still feel like the luckiest man around" (Lustbader, 2001, p. 94). The need for close emotional support does not diminish with age.

People need people for emotional support. Support is often distinguished between instrumental support (such as cooking, shopping, cleaning, etc.) and emotional support (such as being there to cheer others and bolster them psychologically). One study (Rowe & Kahn, 1998) found that

> it was the frequency of emotional support, not instrumental support, which was the powerful predictor of maintained and even enhanced physical function with age. Just good, old-fashioned talk therapy from friends and loved ones helps to keep the aging body vital . . . [and] can also improve mental performance in older people. (pp. 123, 137)

At a fundamental level, identity is ascribed by others in interaction. Simone de Beauvoir (1972) claims that "[o]ne's life has value so long as one attributes value to the life of others, by means of love, friendship, indignation, compassion" (p. 541). Throughout the transitions and stable periods of older adulthood, however, answers to the question "Who am I going to rely upon or be close to?" may change for some. For others, membership in an extended family or kinship network remains constant through adulthood and older adulthood. Relationships provide the vehicle through which one may feel loved, regarded, respected, needed, connected. A sense of usefulness, whether to the family or the community, of being productive in aiding others to achieve well-being, and of maintaining one's own self-respect and self-efficacy are communicated by others. One cannot conjure these in isolation. Being regarded by others as important to their well-being provides many with a reason for being.

For each older adult, the matter of relationships is different. Gender, marital status, place of residence, and cultural identity all impose significant influences. Kinship networks may include both family members as well as nonrelatives who are considered "family." Both same-sex and opposite-sex relationships provide a "significant other" to both give and need support. But for increasing numbers of single persons, mostly nonminority women, and especially those without children, the probability of having to develop supportive relationships in later life is great. Persons who live in institutional settings, whether nursing homes or assisted-living facilities, may have a community-at-hand from which to draw support but be limited in their ability to make friends outside that community.

But equally influential is a person's propensity to make friends. Some individuals are extroverts, others introverts; some are shy, others are outgoing; some are surrounded, others isolated; some are members of social, family, religious, or cultural groups where it is impossible to be alone, while others have few acquaintances. Professionals and others may be introduced to this task area when relationships go awry, when families and an older loved one are in conflict, when a last support person dies, or when persons are confronted by the virtual absence of support, as in the following instance:

> When retiring from an active legal practice, an attorney became aware that among his clients were a small number for whom he was their only support person or contact. No matter what their need, his was the

number they called. Some lived in their own homes; others were in care facilities. Some had adequate financial resources; others were very limited. All were alone, no family, no friends. This discovery led him to continue his relationship with them. He sees his work now less as a legal counsel and more as a minister and social worker, with a renewed dedication to this client population who have no one else.

Fundamental to living all of one's days is the role played by others. Profound needs are met in these interactions that assume different shapes and significance as the transitions and periods that follow are lived. Fahey and Holstein (1993, p. 243) note that the knowledge of our own finitude makes this "a time of vivid tension between the needs of self and others," a knowledge bound up in the paradox that it is in meeting the needs of others that we meet our own needs.

To Face Loss and Address Change

How does one begin a conversation about a process that will deplete a person's most treasured relationships, abilities, and possessions? Is it framed as a dirge, a warning, an opportunity, or simply as one more occasion for planning? Is the experience of loss or change limited to an individual or a couple, or is it experienced by a family or extended kinship network?

Mary Pipher (1999) described the accumulation of loss this way: "When people are in their thirties, they worry about losing their looks. In their fifties, they worry about losing capacities. By their seventies, people worry about losing everything" (p. 161). And rightly so. The list of losses is long, it is cumulative, and it portends the ultimate. Any discussion of loss in the latter years acknowledges the immanence of one's final and complete loss of life.

Some losses are incremental, commencing years earlier and gradually making their impact felt. Loss of hearing or vision are examples. Losses experienced as the result of discrimination or poverty are also examples. Other losses crash into otherwise peaceful and unsuspecting lives in a moment, without warning, such as a stroke or cancer diagnosis. Such losses are random thieves—no single order, no prescribed time. Some losses are temporary, such as the short-term loss of mobility when recovering from a serious injury. Others are permanent. Many losses are exacerbated when the experience of gender, race, sexual orientation, or class limits the resources and reserves available to confront them. Facing losses requires the support of others, a reason for living, and, often, financial resources. Professionals are frequently involved in situations where resources must be identified and secured to address the needs of those with limited financial and relational resources.

The discharge planning unit of a nearby hospital consists of a nurse and social worker who are frequently confronted with older patients, ready to be released, who live alone, have limited support networks consisting mainly of frail contemporaries, are unable to care for themselves, and haven't the resources to hire care. The nurse and social worker are faced with the dual tasks of locating a secure environment for the patient's recovery and securing the public resources to pay for it.

Professionals and family members are also challenged to support persons and to aid them in developing support networks when a significant loss, such as the death of a spouse or the inability to care for oneself, intrudes. In addition to the instrumental aspects of care and support, there is also the need for moral support and encouragement. These losses may feel overwhelming to the one who experiences them. Often young people speak of being challenged to the core, "to see what we are made of." Older adults are challenged to discern not only their substance but their spirit in the face of loss, and professionals and family members are frequently enlisted to stand with them.

Remarkably, a great many persons remain resilient in old age, and despite the challenges possess a high sense of satisfaction. According to Baltes and Baltes (1990),

Research has yielded counterintuitive evidence on this topic that is critical for an adequate conception of mastery in old age. Because of a negative aging stereotype, one might easily expect that older persons would hold less positive views of themselves and their efficacy to control their own lives. Contradictory to this expectation, however, old people on the average do not differ from young people in reports of their subjective life satisfaction. (p. 18)

But growth out of loss is neither inevitable nor automatic. Lost opportunities are not always the creators of new horizons, nor does stoic acceptance necessarily transform itself into hopeful visions. In many situations, coping equates to steadfast suffering. Baltes and Baltes (1998) assert that "as we move into advanced old age in particular, the central task becomes increasingly one of maintenance and management of losses" (p. 17). In other situations, coping involves specific steps to overcome or to compensate for a loss. Can one do better than balance gains and losses? B. F. Skinner (1983), from the vantage of his own older years, advised that old age be regarded as a problem to be solved (pp. 23-24). Skinner's approach clearly identifies the aging process, replete with losses and variations, as a series of challenges to be faced and overcome.

Moving beyond suffering and acceptance to look loss in the eye, older persons can pursue new purposes, embrace new values, adopt new habits, accept new responsibilities, develop new relationships, and thereby re-create themselves and be stronger, wiser, and more mature from the experience. Poet Paul Claudel, at 80, captured this determination in writing: "No eyes left, no ears, no teeth, no legs, no wind! And when all is said and done, how astonishingly well one does without them!"* (cited in Fahey and Holstein, 1993, p. 245).

A word about change: Compared with the devastation of loss, change might seem little more than an irritation. Although some changes are made voluntarily (sometimes at the urging of family members or professionals), other changes happen outside of one's control and may represent a loss of the way things were. These may include changes in the environment ("the neighborhood has changed"), changes in organizations ("the new pastor never seems to remember my name"), changes in social networks ("I have no one to call since Nettie died"), changes in resources ("things got really tight when my son lost his job"), or changes in the family ("the grandchildren's activities seem to rule out frequent visits"), resulting in a change in one's place in the overall scheme of things. Some changes may have positive aspects hidden within them: the death of a spouse may bring the badly needed insurance money; or decline in mobility may result in a move from the large family home that required extensive maintenance to more manageable housing; or a loss of health may result in closer and more frequent attention from one's family.

---

*From *Voices and Visions of Aging: Toward a Critical Gerontology,* edited by T.R. Cole, W.A. Ashenbaum, P.O. Jakobi, & R. Kastenbaum, © 1993. Reproduced with permission of Springer Publishing Company, LLC, New York, NY 10036.

Change and loss often merge into varied shapes. As one moves ahead through the stages of development, priorities are reframed and tasks and activities necessary in an earlier stage, but no longer appropriate, are left behind, often with reluctance or even pain, a way of life gone forever. One is faced with changes that are difficult but possible, as in a lifestyle, and with changes about which one can do little or nothing, as in health or mobility. Both discomfort and irritate. Like loss, change can provide the setting for planning, problem solving, and doing what is necessary to create meaning and thereby re-create the self.

CONCLUSION

As persons age, the years behind them become larger and more consuming. By implication, their present is valuable only as it is enfolded into the past. A pernicious ethos in many communities of older adults defines people by what they once were. For example, a friend retired in the 1960s from his position as paymaster of a large New York corporation and relocated to a community in the Southwest. A visit decades later showed him still identified in the community's directory only by who he was as a professional years earlier, implying that residents are no more than what they once were. This view is also reflected in obituaries that chronicle a person's life until retirement and then skip to the cause of death. This book is about an older adult's present and future, and the inherent tasks related to purpose, autonomy, relationships, and changes and losses.

A focus on a future potent enough to escape the domination of the past requires examination of the structure and tasks of the years ahead. Is it too ambitious to suggest that persons be encouraged to plan to live all of their days? To refuse to give up one whit of joy or fulfillment from the final years? To decline to waste any human potential derived from the time and experience of any older person? The tasks stand as agenda for the future, describing the process of personal re-creation, of contributing to society, and of satisfying hopes and desires, in other words, describing a complete life.

Carl Klaus (1999) in *Taking Retirement* describes how colleagues planted a young tree in his honor in a park near his home. Each day as he watched it he wondered whether he, like the tree, was growing and thriving. The latter years are clearly capable of being such a time.

Chapter 2

Entering Older Adulthood

How does one arrive at older adulthood? Is there an observable point of entry into the latter years, a single line that all must cross? Do all persons experience a single rite of passage? Professionals who serve older adults are confronted with several gateways by which persons currently enter older adulthood, some widely recognized in the popular culture, others more subtle and much less noticed.

RETIREMENT

The most common gateway in the popular imagination is the transition from the world of work called retirement, in which one discontinues the full-time employment that has provided a livelihood through the adult years and negotiates a path into a new life-world. Retirement as it is presently understood is a comparatively recent idea: Formerly, only the wealthy could afford to discontinue work. In earlier centuries, few lived much beyond the end of their work lives, and, consequently, there were few "retirement years" to consider. People simply continued doing what they had always done, often at a reduced pace, or turned to work that was less demanding. When they finally could no longer work, they lived on their savings or depended on their children or neighbors.

Currently, retirement is an available gateway to those who have been employed during a significant portion of their adulthood and who can afford financially to discontinue that employment and be supported by pensions, Social Security, and other financial resources.

A Journey Called Aging: Challenges and Opportunities in Older Adulthood
© 2007 by The Haworth Press, Taylor & Francis Group. All rights reserved.
doi:10.1300/5915_03

Until relatively recently, retirement was a phenomenon quite widely associated with persons who were members of the working classes, the middle classes, and above. However, as many companies have shifted from defined benefit pension plans to 401(k) plans, many workers find that their savings are not sufficient to support retirement without paid work—the average 401(k) holds only $39,600. The number of older retirees returning to work is growing quickly. In a recent study, about one-third of those returning to work said they needed the extra income to survive financially (Bernasek, 2006).

The word *retirement* is generally used in two ways: to refer to the process of retiring and to the whole period of life after one has ceased working at what was one's highest status, highest paying employment. Clarity about this usage may come from comparing retirement with graduation. Graduation has a before, a during, and an after: the years of school, "the big day" itself, and the months afterward where one moves from student status to full-fledged membership in the adult working population. Retirement as a transition also has a before, a during, and an after. The before is the lifetime of work. The during involves the decision to quit, the process of arranging for an orderly departure, with appropriate financial planning, and the single day when, perhaps with a celebratory luncheon, depending on the worker's status, one turns in one's keys or one's final timecard and leaves for the last time. The after is the time it takes to get from the status of worker to a rhythm of life that has its own integrity, goals, commitments, and schedule as an older adult. Retirement, the transition from work to nonwork, in its most intense form, usually occurs within the space of a year or so.

Professor Joseph F. Quinn (2001) of Boston College broadens this picture:

> For many Americans, retirement is not an event, but rather a process that involves, over time, departure from a career job, the receipt of Social Security and employer pensions benefits, some transitional employment, and eventually complete labor force withdrawal. Where along this exit route one is defined as "retired" is much less important than understanding the steps and their determinants along the way. (p. 126)

TIME OF RETIREMENT

The age of 65 has been associated with retirement because until recently it was the age when one could get full Social Security benefits, although during the past half century the age at which older Americans retire has been decreasing. In 1950, 83.4 percent of men aged 55 to 64 were employed; by 1990, only 67.8 percent of men in this age group were working (U.S. Department of Commerce, 1953, p. 185; 1996, p. 393). The influx of women into the labor market resulted in participation rates for women that were steady during the post–World War II period, but which during the 1980s began to increase significantly (Quinn, 2001, p. 125). In 1999, 58.6 percent of workers elected to receive Social Security benefits at age 62, the earliest age at which those benefits became available to them (U.S. House of Representatives, 2000, Section 1, Tables 1-14).

"I didn't choose age. It chose me. And here I am," confessed a friend, beginning his search for a way through this time of life. This friend chose early retirement after having been diagnosed with a potentially terminal disease. He decided to stop work in order to enjoy his remaining years. Many others in good health and with sufficient resources have made the same choice for the same reason.

As a result, according to Murray Gendell (2000), when comparing the average age of retirement with expected longevity,

> the duration of men's retirement increased from 12 years in 1950-55 to 17.4 years in 1990-1995. This gain of 5.4 years expanded men's retirement by 45 percent. The comparable change for women was from 13.6 years to 21.1 years, a rise of 55 percent. Thus, over the 40 years period since the early 1950s, the duration of retirement grew in the United States by about 50 percent. (p. 7)

At the same time, the number of Americans over 65 who work has been rising since the mid-1990s, and in 2000, the 12.8 percent of older adults in the workforce was higher than at any time since 1979, but much lower than 50 years ago (Walsh, 2001). One factor already mentioned is the need for some older persons to work to survive financially. Factors that prompt older persons to seek employment include reductions in medical insurance for retirees; changes in many retirement pension programs and limitations on benefits; the anticipation of increased health and longevity that may mean that some seniors will outlive their financial resources; and the present reality that the cost of living without a regular income is greater than the available resources.

Another factor often mentioned is the need for older persons in the workplace. In some instances, demographic cycles leading to diminished numbers of younger age workers direct employers to an older adult population to fill shortages in the labor force. In other instances, employers seek to hire (or rehire) older workers because of their particular expertise or their reputation for reliability and loyalty. Changes in federal legislation that abolished mandatory retirement for most workers and changes in Social Security rules have encouraged and rewarded continued work by adults beyond the ages at which they formerly might have retired, in contrast to earlier policies that tended to deter such employment.

Thus, the total picture paradoxically includes both an increasing number who choose to retire at an age earlier than 65 as well as an increasing number who choose to continue to work past the age of 65.

POSTRETIREMENT EMPLOYMENT

For reasons mentioned, definitions of retirement are expanding. Although traditionally based on labor force withdrawal, more recent definitions, recognizing continued employment of some sort, have included receipt of retirement benefits such as Social Security and pensions as well. Therefore, persons may be judged to be retired either because they have ceased work or because they are receiving retirement benefits.

The trend toward "postretirement employment" takes many forms. Obviously, some employed persons simply maintain and continue their careers until an advanced age, with or without retirement or any job modification. For others, it takes the form of part-time or flexible-time work, either with the former employer, or in a new area of employment altogether. It may also take the form of phased retirement in which the worker systematically transitions out of a position over several years with an increasingly reduced workload. According to Anna M. Rappaport (2001), "[f]ew employers offer formal programs to accommodate gradual retirement in their companies, so phased retirement is usually achieved through a bridge job" (p. 1). A bridge job is defined as a short-term job after retiring from a career in contrast to a career job that lasts ten years or more. More than a third of Americans have a bridge job before leaving the labor force entirely (Rappaport, 2001, p. 6). Self-employment at either part- or full-time status also may serve to take the place of earlier paid full-time employment.

A newspaper reporter for a metropolitan daily, tired of her job and the new assignments imposed by her employer, gave up writing columns at age 65, collected her benefits, and became a part-time "hired pen" for several local firms and an active community volunteer. A cardiologist resigned her full-time position at a medical clinic and began a part-time research project for a local medical college, expecting the part-time responsibility to phase out her employment. A professor agreed to reduce his teaching load by 25 percent each year in order to phase in his retirement over four years. Some in the business world reduce their responsibility over time, and others transition into self-employment in a variety of roles from consultants to home improvement specialists.

> Upon retirement, a maintenance worker at a local industry secured a position with his small municipality conducting daily tests of the drinking water in that village and trouble-shooting problems with the water distribution system. He relished the position, saying that it was the best job he had ever had because it allowed discretionary use of his time, provided some income, and made him a highly valued member of the community: when there were problems with the water, people always called him.

Others may choose to continue activities formerly connected with their paid employment, but without remuneration. A market researcher continued to use his surveying skills in the new community to which he retired, providing a critical impetus to the economic development program getting underway. Barbara Meyerhoff (1978) shares the insight of a retired tailor:

> I'm doing what I have always done. My thinking hasn't changed, so my attitude hasn't changed. You could say I'm still working. Am I retired now because nobody pays me for this? The only thing that happened was when I was sixty-five I took off my watch. (p. 46)

In tracking the retirement patterns of CEOs and other high-ranking business executives, Jeffrey Sonnenfeld (1988) discovered that many retired chief executives denied that they had "really retired" and wanted to be recognized as busy and important people (p. 12). He concluded that retirement was a difficult transition for this population because their own purpose and self-worth were strongly linked to the well-being of the firms of which they were leaders. Upon retirement, the chief executive is "suddenly left without a ready personal identity, for the work-intensive executive does not see a job as a mere form of livelihood, but as an extension of his or her self-concept" (p. 57). One of Sonnenfeld's case study subjects describes the loss of identity as moving from "who's who" to "who's he" (p. 213). He observes:

> Sometimes retirement provides the leader with an opportunity to prove his heroic potential to himself, as well as to others, by rising above it, perhaps by seeking a new community where he can promote his vision and reconfirm his self-image. (p. 57)

At the other end of the economic continuum is another population unable to retire:

> Will describes himself as a handyman. Since adolescence, he has worked for others doing home maintenance tasks, ranging from carpentry to painting and landscaping. He uses his old truck to haul salvaged building materials. Steady employment was frequently interrupted by health problems as well as by the availability of clients able to pay for his services. As a self-employed businessperson, he was never able to set aside funds for a retirement pension or savings. Now that he is an older adult, he finds that he must continue to ply his trade in order to contribute to the economy of his extended family.

According to the U.S. Census Bureau (2003b), 10.1 percent of all persons over the age of 65 live below poverty level. However, for older African Americans, that proportion increased to 21.9 percent, compared with whites at 8.1 percent, and others, including Hispanics, Native Americans, and Asian Americans, at 17.7 percent.

Recent income studies of people over 65 reveal some quite startling facts about the importance of Social Security for half the population over age 65. According to a Congressional Research Service report cited in *Aging Today*, for "the lowest quartile of elders in the

United Sates, those with incomes of less than $9,390 in 2004, Social Security provided 86 percent of their total income on average. The third quartile, people with incomes from $9,390 to $15,199, depended on Social Security for 82 percent of their incomes." The report goes on to note that "[f]ifty-six percent [of Americans age 65 and over] received income from assets, such as stocks, bonds, checking accounts and savings. Average income from this source was $5,374, and the median was $95" (Rosenblatt, 2006, p. 2).

The need for postretirement employment as well as the need to delay the time of retirement may depend to a large part on a person's economic well-being as measured by assets such as Social Security benefits, savings and pensions, home ownership, and health insurance. However, choices concerning postretirement employment are also influenced by other important factors: the interest and expertise of the person, the work conditions and flexibility of the position, causes or activities that compete for attention, plus the anticipation of decades of longevity ahead. Work has also become a default option for those unable to discover fulfilling roles in retirement. It should be clear that there is no single normative script that is universally followed. The means and style of entry from work into older adulthood differ, not only at any point in time, but also over time, as employers' needs for workers and older adults' needs for financial support and creative activity take different shapes and assume greater or lesser importance.

> Jennie and Dean both retired, she from a secretarial position, he from work on an assembly line. Plans for living on their small savings and retirement income were disrupted by the need for significant financial support for their children and grandchildren. So before the ink on their retirement documents had time to dry, both had secured other positions. Jennie is the program coordinator for a nonprofit organization, and Dean is with a small company, assembling motors. As their health has declined, the health insurance programs provided by their new employers have made it necessary for one of them to continue to work.

Scenarios differ, but common elements persist: dominant is the need to "make ends meet." For some, this need represents a continuation in a lifetime of poverty; but for others, it means securing the resources to live as one chooses. A second element is the desire to escape boredom by having a regularly scheduled activity. For increasing numbers, work is the answer to the question "What shall I do?"

Some greet retirement warmly; others are thrust into it. For many, it is the result of decades of planning and saving, but for others, it occurs in sudden and unexpected ways. Some may approach this transition as a simple change, others as a crisis. And many confess that the process didn't happen exactly as they had planned. The markers of a transition—cessation, change, discontinuity, uncertainty, anomie, perhaps some chaos—all may apply, depending on the individual's circumstance and perspective.

Professionals may discover many instances where older adults work either full-time or part-time in order to survive financially. Employment is clearly an economic necessity for increasing numbers of older persons. This is true both of persons with low incomes and of those unable to avoid living beyond their means. But it would be a mistake to assume that money is always the motivator, or the only motivator. Careful planning for the present and the future requires understanding all of the reasons why a person returns to work: these include having an identity or status, having something to do each day, and having colleagues with whom to do it, as well as the need for monetary resources. Helping older people to plan for the present and future should focus on what to live for as well as what to live on.

RETIREMENT VARIATIONS

Poverty as a fact of life encourages many to continue employment. But according to Ryff and others (Ryff, Magee, Kling, & Wing, 1999, p. 258), "a growing body of evidence links socioeconomic standing to a diverse array of health outcomes." That is, poverty has adverse health consequences (p. 259), and it imposes a greater risk of occupational injury (Stoller & Gibson, 2000, p. 127). Both factors combine to explain a higher level of disability among the poor and working classes, many of whom are members of minority groups. For those who are unable to work because of physical impairment, permanent disability serves as an alternative to retirement.

Katherine lives alone in a central city subsidized apartment. She refused to give her age, but she admitted to working past the age when many people retire; furthermore, she has taken advantage of senior programs for over a decade. Her six children are scattered across the country, two living in the same city as their mother. All check in by telephone nearly every day. To support her family, Katherine worked as a household assistant until an injury forced her to discontinue employment. She describes how she managed the households of some wealthy citizens; however, only in the last few years did her employers participate in the Social Security program. Therefore, her small Social Security check requires additional Supplemental Security Income (SSI). For medical care, she relies on a Medicaid card. Back pain has continued to plague her to the point that on some days she has difficulty getting around. But everyone in the building knows Katherine, and Katherine knows everyone. The same is true in her church. When asked about her future plans, or what will happen when she can no longer live independently, Katherine says simply, but with conviction, "The Lord will provide."

Katherine has lived a lifetime on the rough edge of poverty. Lack of education, limited employment opportunities, racial discrimination, and the need to support her six children as a single parent have all played a role in determining her present situation as well as her future. Although she carries the demeanor of an independent person, Katherine is surrounded by an active church community as well as by a caring family. She believes this strong support postpones critical decisions about living alone. Retirement came only when she was unable to continue working.

Another variation on the retirement theme occurs with workers who in their fifties lose their employment as the result of a corporate downsizing, a change in the business cycle, or when a business moves to another location. Some organizations provide "outplacement counseling" and other services designed to help secure another position. But many, after joining the ranks of the unemployed, find it difficult to secure a new position at a level similar to their former job. When they reach the age at which pension or Social Security benefits may be accessed, unemployment is transmuted into retirement.

A purchasing manager, laid off because he was "redundant" in a corporate merger, learned to his disappointment that there was no market for a person of his age and skills. He converted unemployment into retirement—a forced choice. Others come to retire unexpectedly as well as reluctantly: they are presented early retirement benefits that may not be welcome, but that must be accepted. Whether termed a "retirement package," "severance pay," or "bridge income," it serves to provide support between the discontinuation of salary and the beginning of pension and Social Security benefits, and whether generous or limited, it often represents an employee's initiation into retirement.

OTHER GATEWAYS

Many studies indicate that unmarried older women are less likely than either unmarried older men or older couples to have savings and financial reserves adequate to support them in older adulthood. In fact, about 20 percent of single older women compared with 6 percent of older couples live in poverty, and 30 percent of black women age 65 and over and 25 percent of Hispanic women, compared with 11 percent of white women over age 65, live in poverty (U.S. House of Representatives, 2000, Appendix A, Table A-6).

The decrease in the median income of the population over 65 can be associated with differences in marital status, since the decrease is due in part to the disproportionate number of unmarried women in older age groups (Social Security Administration, 2003). Consequences of widowhood or divorce among many older women include both diminished economic status and reduced social status and identity, introducing the necessity for them to participate in employment past the typical retirement age.

> Ruth, a widow in her early seventies, lives in a nice apartment on the edge of the business district in a small city. While her family was together, she was a stay-at-home mom. After the children left the nest and her husband died, she obtained employment as a clerk in a local card and stationery store. Her children argue that she shouldn't have to work, and that her limited income is adequate to support her. She listens politely, knowing that she couldn't afford all of the things she enjoys without that income, and affirms that she has no intention of quitting her job: "What would I do if I didn't work?"

Retail establishments, fast-food restaurants, and other low-wage service industries employ large numbers of part-time and full-time older workers, in many instances women and persons of color who are required to supplement their limited financial resources and benefits.

Women who experience either divorce or widowhood during their adult years may be vulnerable to the unanticipated loss of financial support that they had counted on for their older years (Walker, Manoogian-O'Dell, McGraw, & White, 2001, p. 180).

> Dolly, now in her mideighties and in good health, lost her husband a year after his retirement. They had no children, and she was never employed outside the home. Upon his death, his pension terminated, as did the supplementary health insurance. For the past twenty years, she has continued to live in their modest suburban home, with Social Security as her only source of income. Dolly is careful to take advantage of programs designed to assist low-income seniors in upgrading her appliances and performing home maintenance. She has cultivated relationships with two neighbors who assist her with tasks she is unable to perform alone. In return, she looks after their homes while they are away and stops by occasionally with home-baked goods. She says frequently that without their assistance she would not be able to stay in her own home.

Dolly and her husband didn't plan for this outcome of a life together. More careful planning might have included a savings account, life insurance, and a continuation of his pension over a longer period. His unexpected death left her to make the best of their limited resources. Her own planning for the short term focuses mainly on stretching the Social Security check to meet all of her needs. Beyond that, she wonders what she will do when she will no longer be able to remain in her home. Although Dolly operates her finances on a razor-thin margin and has little family to support her, she has a number of resources: the equity in her home, the support of neighbors, and her own good health and determination.

Contrast Dolly's situation with that of Josephine:

> Josephine is the unemployed mother of Gary, a developmentally disabled son on public assistance. As his only caregiver, she has transitioned from one form of government support to another, carrying both her poverty and her responsibility with her into the third age. Her entry into older adulthood has gone unnoticed, since little has changed, except that she qualifies for different benefits.

In this instance, a professional is challenged at several levels: to help a person survive economically, to help plan goals and activities meaningful to the persons involved, and to help plan for the care and maintenance of the son after Josephine is no longer able, or present, to do so.

The perception of entry into older adulthood captured in the simple image of an employee making a clean and abrupt break from employment clearly does not apply to all. For some, the gateway involves the conclusion of the work of a spouse, and for others, it involves movement into older adulthood by dint of public markers, such as claiming Social Security benefits. One can, of course, also come to this transition simply by living long enough.

WHAT ABOUT HOMEMAKERS?

Those who have not experienced employment outside of the home, such as traditional homemakers, have entered this period by virtue of their own years or by virtue of the retirement of their spouses. One homemaker reported she saw no major changes in her responsibility after her husband stopped work in his sixties. She appreciated the newfound flexibility in his schedule, his availability to be helpful around the house, and their freedom to travel in ways not possible before he stopped working. A recently widowed person said that her husband's insurance money would now make it possible for her to enjoy retirement.

The transition into older adulthood is often more difficult to see clearly in the case of women who have been lifelong homemakers. For many, there seems to be no retirement, no change, no release from homemaking tasks, but a period replete with continued responsibility. Although many homemakers do not retire, they nevertheless enter older adulthood by virtue of their age and their receipt of Social Security.

This was particularly true for women in Fisher's (1993) study who had been homemakers and caregivers through most of their adulthood and for whom retirement was a particularly elusive concept. For those who worked as homemakers and caregivers at home, retirement from work did not have a distinct date and appeared to occur later than for the spouse who worked outside the home. One woman was typical in her response: "I never worked outside the home, so I didn't have any plans for retirement." Another said, "I've never retired. I'm always working in the house."

Several said that in retirement they had less work to do because they didn't have the responsibility of children, giving them more time for themselves. Another said her routine changed greatly when her husband retired.

Women who had not been employed outside the home usually continued their homemaking activities until unable to do so. One woman complained that she hoped that after she had worked hard all of her life, she would have some relief in retirement, but she was disappointed:

> I still have to work hard. I still have to take care of myself. I'm still walking. I always wished for a car and still don't have one. I thought I could go places and do things, but I can't. I cook, paint, clean, sew, do washing. When you don't have anything, and everybody has something, you hope that someday the time will come that it'll be that way for you.

This woman's complaint is that nothing has changed. The poverty with which she had struggled throughout adulthood continues to surround her. She sees others for whom older adulthood provides something of a respite and mourns that it is not so for her. The hope for a better life for herself does not terminate with entry into older adulthood.

This woman represents others who enter older adulthood carrying the burden of home care and significant caregiving responsibilities that, combined with the lack of adequate financial resources, can cast a dark shadow over these years. Opportunities to escape lifelong responsibility, whether at home or in a position outside the home, are diminished, particularly among women and minorities and among all whose limited resources restrict their options. At the same time, women who find their traditional homemaking roles the source of fulfillment persist in continuing those activities and responsibilities that have defined them over their adulthood.

The response of professionals to situations in which persons entering older adulthood lack resources, whether financial or personal support, varies, depending on the nature of the situation, on the particular professional specialty involved, and on the professional's view of the role of a professional. In some instances, professionals are able to assist the person to change the situation by identifying and securing the kinds of assistance needed to address some, if not all, of the problems involved. In other instances, the professional's role is seen, not as one of changing a situation, but as one of assisting the older person to adapt to that situation.

THE CORE

The transition into older adulthood may vary among individuals in several respects. For some, its common center is the transition from the world of work into a world after work; for others, it represents a significant change or diminution within the world of work; and for still others, the transition into older adulthood is marked by the accumulation of years, the receipt of retirement benefits, plus the myriad changes—physical and social—that tend to accompany this entry. It may be a carefully orchestrated process, planned by the participant and occurring on schedule, or it may be as unexpected as a notice to clean out one's desk by a certain time tomorrow, or as traumatic as hearing a physician say that one has less than a year to live. It may be an orderly transition—all of the components in position—or it may consist of random elements that refuse to fall neatly into place. It may be surgically clean, or it may carry some unfinished business of pre-transitional activities. Bridge, phased, or other employment commitments may blur the distinction between before and after. The emotions associated with the transition may likewise range from great excitement to deep disappointment to sheer ennui, and their intensity, from "business as usual" to "this is the end."

For some, it is welcome to be relieved of responsibility, to have more control over their time, and to choose how to make use of their energy. This is the time for which many have worked and saved, the time awaited from the first paycheck deduction for Social Security benefits, an anticipation that may have increased over time. Others believe a giant black hole filled with the nothingness of inactivity awaits them. Others may scarcely have noticed the change.

But while the pathways and emotions may vary, the central theme of the embarkation into older adulthood for a majority of persons is that one moves from a life's work into a period of indeterminate length without a culturally sanctioned agenda, and where choices await regarding use of time and resources, purpose for living, and relationships to be nurtured. In the case of members of ethnic or culturally delineated groups, there are traditions defining the role and status of older persons that continue to voice the group's expectations. For homemakers, chances are that much of their lifelong agenda operates in older adulthood much as before, unless they are able, with or without the help of professionals, family, or friends, to change the expectations of their roles in older adulthood held by others as well as themselves. Although the transition into older adulthood is usually relatively brief, no one can predict how long older adulthood will last for any individual, creating both uncertainty and difficulty in planning.

Many have described their surprise at the unexpected scope of the transition. Nancy Schlossberg (2004) says of her own experience:

> The ease of letting go of a past role depends on the degree to which it was central to your identity. Clearly, my role as a professor of counseling psychology was central to my sense of self. Letting go of that, and having nothing to do, created a vacuum. Friends warned me that I would flunk retirement. . . .
>
> The vacuum is a period of neither-here-nor-there, during which you are relinquishing one set of roles, relationships, routines, and assumptions, and struggling to figure out "what next." (pp. 18, 19)

Another professional related his experience of the first year after he retired:

> I quickly learned that being busy and being productive were not the same. Setting priorities was a challenge. Going with the flow and allowing environment and circumstance to manage my life was an inviting temptation. The word best describing what I learned during that first year is "initiative." Purpose needed choosing, friends called, activities selected, and a future planned.

The uncharted path, the blank slate, and a host of surprises underline the need to identify next steps in enriching one's life during the ensuing years. The research upon which this book is based presents a map to clarify the direction and guide the journey over the road ahead. It may mean surprise, both in what greets the traveler on this road and in what is absent. But any traveler who believes that the choices and decisions awaiting are easy and without stress should be reminded that the words *travel* and *travail* come from the same root. Counseling professionals with particular knowledge of the retirement transition can help ease the difficulty of this adjustment. Symptoms of the difficulties in adjusting may appear in many other areas, such as physical and mental health, relationships, and finances. Professionals who address only the symptoms may miss underlying causes.

MOVING OUT, LETTING GO

During the adult years, life circumstances, employment, and family and community obligations all contributed to the view of what life was about. They structured life. Their agenda provided meaning. The people at home and the people at work made relationships happen. There was a great security in a lifestyle whose structure, meaning, and relationships were self-evident, if not stable. But in retiring, the interplay of employment and family have changed—employment no longer shapes life's purpose as it once did, while relationships may take on more importance.

Robert S. Weiss (2005) concludes his fascinating study of the transition from work to retirement with these observations about what he learned:

Retirement means changing how one relates to the social world. It means leaving a career, a community of work, and a way of life. It is likely to bring with it extraordinary freedom. It may also expose the retiree to social isolation. . . .

More of an immediate concern [than finances] for many retirees is the impact on them of the loss of their community of work. Some degree of social isolation can be inescapable in the short run for retirees who have no other community membership with which to replace their membership in the community of work. . . .

There are many forms of activity available to the retired, each with its own mix of contribution and constraints. . . .

Perhaps most important for the quality of life in retirement is the retiree's relationship with his or her life partner. As couples move toward retirement their marriages change from partnerships in the management of home and family to companionships. More time is likely to be spent together. Retirement then provides still more time together. Being able to enjoy that additional time together can decide whether the retirement will be gratifying or burdensome. (pp. 178-179)

One should not underestimate the task of separating oneself from an employment community and purpose that have been consuming over the years and have provided a home. Nancy Schlossberg (2004) asks, "How will I live without applause? We all love to be noticed, recognized, and made to feel we matter. 'Applause' is a metaphor for this kind of reinforcement which, ideally, we received from our work" (p. 32). The transition itself has been filled with separation; it is not surprising that separation anxiety can result. Nor should one underestimate the sheer relief that some feel when, finally, they are freed from a job they did mainly for the money. But for them, too, the separation is real and the feelings surrounding it can be more than trivial.

The same sort of separation anxiety may be present in other roles as well. For some, the continuation of adult roles into older adulthood may be a matter of necessity or of conscious choice. For others, homemakers, for example, tasks like food preparation have about them such a comfortable familiarity that it is difficult for many to even think of giving it up voluntarily or living without it. Separation from such roles, as in the case of separation from employment, can be the source of considerable anxiety.

More serious than the separation is the transition into something—but what? Is there a person who doesn't remember with some feeling the anxiety of adolescence? It was a time of excitement, filled with mixed signals about expectations. One moment it said, "Be an adult!" Next it said, "You are only a child." An adolescent walks the fine line between childhood and adulthood, aspiring to adult activities but able to take refuge in youthful years. It was a time of experimenting with various roles and responsibilities of the grown-up, without really being an adult.

Into this mix of childhood and adulthood came the persistent questions, "What do you want to be when you grow up?" and "What do you want to do for a living?" The burdens of being and doing were imposed, expecting wise choices, setting direction, developing plans, learning how to be the person chosen, and all the rest. A second question accompanied the first, "With whom will you do it?" Choices of purpose were accompanied by the choices for significant relationships. Addressing tasks defining identity and intimacy, according to Erik Erikson (1950), provided the framework for the choices of adolescence.

In adolescence, choices were made for an adulthood yet to be experienced. In contrast, the choices that introduce older adulthood proceed from a lifetime of knowledge, experience, and more or less already formed and wise opinions. True, at the moment of decision, there may be limited experience of retirement or old age. But there is the experience of adulthood with its multiple roles of citizen, taxpayer, employee, volunteer, family member, friend, and person. And there is, almost certainly, the experience of grieving a lost relationship or role, and moving on. The years flesh out the emotional, spiritual, cultural, and environmental dimensions of the experience of adulthood in a tapestry of lived experience that provides the backdrop for choices about the next years.

But middle age provides minimal experience of aging, often limited to observations of aging parents. Some experiences show a negative side of aging, as when an older relative has lived in our home while being cared for during periods of illness or disability. Certainly the vicarious experience that comes from the media, literature, and culture is seldom adequate preparation for one's own aging.

Thus, in the transition into older adulthood, the questions that had such urgency at the end of adolescence recur—namely, identity and intimacy. To them is joined the question of generativity: "What are you going to do that makes a difference?" The answers to these three questions—in short-hand, "Who am I? What am I going to do? With whom am I going to do it?"—will structure the successful completion of the transition or retiring.

For some, those choices have been revisited periodically throughout adulthood. Levinson and colleagues (1996, 1978) suggest that the men and women studied reexamined their choices and adjusted life accordingly about every ten years. To those who have experienced crises—both major and minor—in midlife, or who have wrestled either by choice or by circumstance with the questions of purpose and relationship, the choices that come at the beginning of older adulthood may not be so different. To them, it may appear to be one more situation where familiar decisions are revisited. For those whose life circumstances have neither prompted nor required revisiting the choices made at adolescence, the segue out of employment may present steeper challenges. Discovering that decisions made "once and for all" were indeed temporary and lasted only through the adult years may confront the person entering older adulthood with an experience ranging from surprise to shock.

For some, the retirement transition will consist of several attempts to create a new set of roles, relationships, and routines. One retiree said, "I retired three years ago. My plans didn't work out, so I started all over again. It wasn't until the third try that I got it right." "Once the structure is created, it is not cast in stone forever. . . . It is comforting to realize that if one path does not work, there are others, and you can enjoy some new scenery on the way" (Schlossberg, 2004, p. 23).

Considerable research has documented the broad impact of times of social change and unrest. The passage from employment into the older adult years can be just such a time. Peter Jarvis (1989) observes that retirement is an "incomplete ritual" since it provides no structural or ritual way to initiate the retiree into a new status in society and into the new roles attached to it. Jarvis writes specifically of retirement as the entry point for older adulthood. Multiply this one point of entry by the number of different examples in this chapter and the scope of the uncertainty and ambiguity of this transition becomes even greater, revealing a greater lack of structure and widely held expectations than might be evident at first glance. Roles to which adults had become accustomed may no longer exist for them, and new roles, clouded by confusion and uncertainty, have yet to be discovered by them. The absence of cultural norms about what is successful aging, or good retirement, or normative older adult behavior serves to enhance the critical nature of the questions revisited from adolescence, about purpose and relationships, and provides a significant level of freedom in discerning the answers. *A Journey Called Aging* endeavors to explore the structure and dynamic of this new landscape of older adulthood.

THE CHALLENGE OF LOOKING AHEAD

With the advent of older adulthood, the challenges of living emerge in greater importance: to discover purpose, to build relationships, to balance autonomy with independence, and to face loss and address change. Mary Pipher (1999) summarizes the situation:

> We humans actually have a fairly small and elemental set of needs. Our surface structures are very different, but all have the same deep structure. We want to be loved, respected, and useful. We want to have fun, and we want to develop our talents. The resilient old have relationships, ways to be useful in their communities, ways to relax, ways to develop their potential, and ways to feel respected. (p. 248)

It takes sensitivity and self-knowledge to walk with patience and understanding alongside someone who is going through difficult transitions. For the professional helper who personally fears the transitions of older adulthood, this will be particularly so. Those who count older adults as patients, clients, colleagues, family members, and friends will discover that despite the experience and maturity gained in adulthood, the needs and challenges present at the beginning of older adulthood are born in a new context, one filled with both apprehension of change and vision of an uncharted future. And as in the launching of any once-in-a-lifetime experience, the embarkation into older adulthood requires support and empathy, sometimes tempered with patience, but always filled with understanding.

Chapter 3

Extended Middle Age

As individuals embark on older adulthood—whether through retirement or by another gateway or by dint of age—they enter upon
a period called Extended Middle Age. The key notion is that of continuity: Extended Middle Age continues the middle age lifestyle and
carries it forward through whatever gateway a person enters older
adulthood.

Extended Middle Age is a stable period; that is, while it has its own
challenges, vibrancy, disappointments, hurts, and gains, it has a core
consistency that gives it an integrity of its own. In Levinson's (1986)
language, it is a time of structure building and life enhancing. It begins at the gateway into older adulthood and ends with the intrusion
of life-changing events, such as the onset of debilitating ill health for
oneself or one's spouse, a significant decrease in physical capability,
the need to relocate, a voluntary major change in lifestyle, or the death
of a spouse.

LENGTH OF DAYS

Extended Middle Age is of indeterminate length: it can be as short
as a few months or as long as a decade or more, depending on the time
of a person's entry into older adulthood. The indeterminate length of
Extended Middle Age can be unnerving for persons used to organizing their lives in terms of a mostly unexamined expectation that next
year will arrive as surely as this one did. It becomes increasingly clear
that persons have very little information about how long they will live
or where the "break points" will come in terms of health and fortune.

A Journey Called Aging: Challenges and Opportunities in Older Adulthood
© 2007 by The Haworth Press, Taylor & Francis Group. All rights reserved.
doi:10.1300/5915_04

At the beginning of or even during Extended Middle Age no one can predict how long this stable period will last. Thus, chronology is no longer the kind of measure it was earlier in life when one had a pretty clear idea of what health and functional ability would be at 30 or 40 or 50. Now, chronology only tells how many years there have been since birth. It does not give us as many clues about health, ability, functions, roles, and relationships as it had seemed to earlier in life. For example, identical twins aged 73 can both be normal in their life course, yet one could be in a health care facility with a degenerative disease that requires care while her sister could be placing well in her age group in the Boston marathon, with her husband cheering her on. A visit to one's fiftieth high school reunion will doubtless reveal, among a population of older adults nearly the same age, some who are in the prime of middle-age fitness and others who are wheelchair bound or require assistance in getting around. In addition to genetic heritage and major life events, the accumulation of diverse life experiences combined with different lifestyles also accounts for increasing contrasts between persons of the same age.

Therefore, as a person proceeds through the gateway into Extended Middle Age, there is a double tension: not knowing how long Extended Middle Age will last, and, as if a harbinger, not knowing how long one's life will last (and therefore—at the simplest level—how one will have to pace the use of time and financial resources in the achievement of one's goals). Carl Klaus (1999, p. 56) writes, "Retirement, after all, is a preparation for other journeys to come, and if I can't adjust to this move, I'll never be able to accept the one that all of us at last are compelled to make."

Middle-Aged Forever

As mortality rates decline among adults, long life becomes more probable, introducing healthy tensions between the need for careful planning on the one hand, and emphasizing the gift of long life on the other. Cusack and Thompson (1999, p. xi) claim that "everyone over fifty strives to stay middle-aged forever." Researchers suggest that this is a good idea: persons over 65 who identify themselves as middle-aged tend to have better adjustment, higher morale, and better health than those who identify themselves as old or elderly (Huyck & Hoyer,

1982, p. 248). They are also more likely to be active and engaged in satisfying activities. Whether the middle-age mind-set brings about those characteristics, or the presence of those characteristics influences the mind-set, the sense of continuation of middle age serves as a positive place from which to begin the older adult experience.

Extended Middle Age is, in the eyes of those living in that period, more closely related to the middle years of life than to the world of older adults. Richard, retired a short time, tells this story:

> A group of retirees went by bus one Wednesday to an art exhibit in a city about 50 miles away. My wife and I decided to join them. We wanted to see the exhibit, and this would save us driving and parking. But when we got on the bus we felt somewhat out of place. Not that these weren't people we recognized. It was just that they were at a stage different from us. They were a "seniors group." It was clear to us that, retired though we were, we were not "seniors."

People in Extended Middle Age look back to the middle years for their self-definition and identification. Could it be that part of the motivation for this direction is to ward off any impending sense of marginalization and to avoid the anticipated deficits that come with advanced age? A view of oneself as middle-aged does not prevent those not yet in the third age from lumping together all people of Social Security or Medicare age. For the cheeky 13-year-old who looks an older person up and down and then says, "So, man, how was Woodstock?" or for the gracious younger woman who offers her seat on the bus, a person's apparent physical age sets one in a poorly refined category of "old." But persons in Extended Middle Age tend to distinguish themselves from other older adults by this sense that they are still middle-aged, and to develop their lifestyles accordingly.

Diversity

According to Fahey and Holstein (1993, p. 244), "the third age is also a time when the cumulative effects of gender, race, and socioeconomic variables, as played out in a strong market economy, are profoundly experienced." For some, these variables portend a level of privilege that comprises retirement from employment, adequate financial and social assets, and opportunities for the interesting and productive use of discretionary time. Some have argued, however, that this image of retirement as the "golden years" is a recent invention, inspired by the marketing efforts of retirement communities and a product of the demographic and economic influences of the last third of the twentieth century. With changing demographics, economics, and lifestyles, some commentators suggest that this image of older adulthood may not be sustainable and may not be the lifestyle of choice for the newest generation to enter older adulthood. It is likely, therefore, that increasing numbers of older adults will combine some levels of employment for compensation with receipt of income from pensions, Social Security, and other retirement plans.

For others, gender, race, and socioeconomic variables restrict choices in an otherwise broad selection of options, imposing conditions that a person cannot control, some caused by the events of adulthood, others by chance, and still others by a person's moment in history. For example, some older adults are still victimized by the poverty that had characterized their middle-age years; the choices available in older adulthood for others, especially in certain ethnic traditions, are engraved in the cultural images of the expected roles of older persons. In addition, structural factors that have negatively affected some minorities—discrimination, unemployment, underemployment, and barriers to health care—may be still in play but may be partially mitigated by social factors, such as the support of families, friends, community, and church, to say nothing of individuals' own cultural and spiritual values (Kiyak & Hooyman, 1994, p. 295).

> After he and his brother decided to "settle out" of the migrant stream in a midwestern city, Fred found a job in a large catalogue warehouse. He did well there until his parents, still living in Texas, became ill. As the oldest, Fred was obliged to make frequent trips to see to their care, causing sporadic absences from work. After he was terminated, he worked during the warm months as a gardener, remembering all that he had learned as a migrant farm worker about the care and nurturing of plants. Fred has continued work as a gardener at several homes and businesses and at other available part-time jobs. Now that he has entered older adulthood, he still feels that he can only lead his family if he is the provider.

The gender variable means, for example, that for every 83 men in the 65 to 74 age group, there are 100 women. A larger proportion of these persons are white (80 percent) than are black, Hispanic, or members of any other racial/ethnic group; 76 percent of men in this age group are married, compared with 52 percent of women; conversely, 30 percent of women are widowed, compared with 8 percent of men. These data play out in the fact that women (and some minorities) tend to have larger support networks than men, and that unmarried persons (as well as those without family, close friends, congregation or group affiliation) experience higher rates of mortality and disease than married persons (Kahn, 1994, p. 164). Associations with older persons, whether as a professional or as a member of this age group, even at this early stage in the older adult life span, will reveal the beginnings of population trends in which the proportions of whites, women, and widows increase in relation to the overall population and in which demographic variables such as gender or marital status are reflected in the diversity of problems and opportunities present in this period.

Approximately 73 percent of the population have graduated high school, and 23 percent of men and 14 percent of women have bachelor's degrees or higher. Conversely nearly a quarter of the population have achieved a lower level of educational attainment; 18 percent of men and 9 percent of women over the age of 65 remained in the labor force in the year 2002. These data translate into various lifestyles, living conditions, opportunities, and income. In 2001, 48 percent of married-couple households over the age of 65 had incomes of $35,000 or more, 31 percent had incomes from $20,000 to $34,999, and 19 percent had incomes of less than $20,000. Approximately 10 percent of families over the age of 65 were below the poverty level in 2001, a proportion that increased for males without wives and increased dramatically for females without husbands (U.S. Census Bureau, 2003c). However, as noted in the introduction, changes are anticipated in women's retirement incomes as women have longer work careers in the future.

Poverty is not the only reason for people to continue to work. A local newspaper recently ran a front-page article about an 85-year-old woman who worked ten hours a day, five days a week, sometimes six, on the assembly line of a small bearing factory and has done so for 35.5 years. Widowed eight years ago, she says, "I get bored if I stay home. Saturday and Sunday, my bones ache more than when I work. It's the exercise of bending and up and down. At home you just sit around" (Dresang, 2005, p. 1). Purpose as well as socialization are strong motivators.

These data present a picture of individuals and families for whom older adulthood represents a continuation of the economic and social patterns established during the adult years. Factors such as gender, marital status, education, employment, health, and ethnic heritage that made a difference in the adult years continue to make a difference in the years after. Within the broad Extended Middle Age experience, these factors still define the options and resources available to individuals.

An Opportunity-Filled Agenda

Extended Middle Age is a time similar to middle age, except that for the large majority of persons, compelling employment obligations are replaced by part-time or sporadic employment, relaxation, sleeping late, travel, and activities ranging from golf to gardening to volunteering. One person marveled at the spirit of the time: "There is nothing you really have to do today."

Freedom has been described as "the most quixotic gift of the third age" (Fahey & Holstein, 1993, p. 244). This statement recognizes that with older adulthood comes release from participation in "the reproductive and productive" systems of society and brings the opportunity to cultivate new personal and social assets. It also comes with a warning that the use of such freedom may stimulate negative responses and personal uncertainty. But it brings the necessary latitude to engage in some degree of personal control.

One aspect of the adaptive process that occurs in Extended Middle Age is the need to participate in a re-creation of the self. For some, re-creation means renewal, the recovery of earlier attributes lost in the adult years. For others, it means the creation of a new identity in place of an identity that may have been appropriate at an earlier age but that no longer works in the opening years of older adulthood. A news article described how persons re-created themselves in retirement: an engineer turned into an inventor, an elementary school teacher became an adult literacy tutor, an executive became an advocate for educational change in her urban school district, a practical nurse became a volunteer for the Red Cross, a full-time professional became a part-time professional, working just when she wants to, and a machinist became a gardener for his church. Many relationships, however, are predicated on one's earlier identity. The process of re-creating the self may test the bounds of one's permission to oneself to consider and implement changes in oneself and in one's relationships with others.

GIVING TIME NEW MEANING

Even with the best planning most will find that the path from planning for older adulthood to a satisfying rhythm of days in Extended Middle Age takes far more intentionality than they anticipate. To the extent that one worked 40+ hours a week, one has now to decide what to do with those 40+ hours. The routine of the work week must be replaced by new ways of using one's time. In Extended Middle Age a significant block of time previously structured by work is now unstructured. In addition to lacking schedule, unstructured time requires that the individual give a new meaning to time—a meaning that is faithful to the self one chooses to be in this part of the journey of life.

This challenge will sit differently with different folks. One fellow noted, "What shocked me was when I realized that every day was unstructured, I no longer had weekends to look forward to." Others have discovered blocks of uninterrupted time that allow for pursuits aimed at reflection, discovering what retirement is for, exploring what one really likes to do, and coming to terms with oneself. Yet others have continued to work and have seen no difference in the balance between work and leisure.

Participation in the workforce declines with age among older adults. Thus, the largest proportion of those engaged in paid employment are in Extended Middle Age. Whether the result of economic necessity, personal preference, opportunities in the workplace, or simply an addiction to professional activity, short-term employment as an integral component of Extended Middle Age has increased during the years since 1995 (Rappaport, 2001). Those with a financial foundation of Social Security and pension benefits may have the luxury of choosing employment for other than economic reasons.

In addition to recasting one's view of time, making space for paid or unpaid work, there is an agenda of adjustment pursuits and activities, indeed of lifestyle, which provides a core for each stable period. Reassessing one's physical and social life space, acknowledging one's limitations, substituting alternative sources of need satisfaction, developing new criteria for self-evaluation, and reintegrating one's values and life goals (Clark & Anderson, 1967) are steps that help a person confront the limitations and opportunities of this new period in ways that bring satisfaction within the constraints of Extended Middle Age. Another way to think of this adjustment process is as the re-creation of oneself in retirement. With the life context changing in each new period, new constraints emerge, inviting new goals and activities, new acceptable levels of achievement, new standards for the good life, and a revised sense of what makes each day worth living. As Nancy Schlossberg (2004, pp. 88-89) notes,

> People take markedly different paths as they structure their lives to obtain the recognition, satisfaction, and meaning they received through work. . . . Retirement is a process in which a retirement career evolves just as a work career did.

An important part of a retirement career is described by Robert Weiss (2005):

> While retirement may mean that our energies or ambitions or zest for work are no longer up to the demands of the work we once did, this says nothing about our wisdom or concern for others or desire to continue to contribute to the social world. . . . Keep time for yourself, yes, but not to the exclusion of continuing to play a role in the world. (p. 191)

Involvement of professionals in the process of adaptation or re-creation often occurs when failure to adapt to new and changing circumstances results in a broad range of symptoms associated with physical or mental health problems, maladaptive personal behavior, or a general sense of life dissatisfaction or malaise. One assembly line worker, upon retirement from an auto manufacturing plant sat in front of the television each day, drinking beer, interrupted only by meals and sleep. Others have responded to retirement with symptoms ranging from severe anxiety to depression. Conversely, many professionals are in a position to observe adaptive behavior as older persons re-create themselves appropriately and with limited stress amid changed circumstances, maintaining a positive outlook, and reaping the benefits in achievement and satisfaction.

Urgency

There is also some sense of urgency to getting on with one's life. Possibly an agenda has developed, consisting of some "retirement goals" or at least some informal ideas in response to the inevitable question "What will you do when you stop work?"

One word of advice came from an older man quite crippled with arthritis, now no longer able to function easily on his own. "Whatever you want to do, do it while you can." The clock is running. Good health and energy and companionship may be running out. The time may come when "you can't do it." There may not be another chance.

This kind of thinking can be helpful in catalyzing people into action. It can also lead a person into thinking of the third age in a two-stage dichotomy: "good years/bad years." As will be clear, this is a false dichotomy. Every period of the third age has its own goals, commitments, promises, dreams, and hopes, to be exercised in the face of its own constraints and burdens. But this sense of urgency points to the fact that most retirement dreams have to do with Extended Middle Age. They assume continuity with the middle years (minus the job). It would be rare, even unthinkable, to hear a retiree respond to the good wishes at a farewell luncheon with sentiments like "When my husband dies, I am planning to . . ." or "I expect to wind up in a fine nursing home . . ." or "When I can't get around without help, my goals are . . ." or "When my kids can no longer take care of me . . ." Clearly most goals for the older years are generated with Extended Middle Age in mind, and bring a sense of urgency to this period.

Goals for Fulfillment

Extended Middle Age can be a time to consider goals that attack the unfinished business accumulated through life, to overcome deficits, to mend fences and renew relationships. Most individuals carry a list headed "I've always wanted to . . ." For them, these years can be catch-up time, now time, fulfillment time.

For example, a surprising number of older persons in adult literacy classes were there because now they had time without the press of work and the obligation of family to complete their high school requirements, or in some cases their elementary school education. These were persons who had worked at positions available to individuals without literacy skills, and whose financial resources were limited. Friends and family occasionally challenged their decision to return to school at this time of life, but throughout adulthood they had promised themselves they would continue their education. One woman found her motivation in a promise she had made on her mother's deathbed that she would get her high school diploma. Now was promise-keeping time. Examples such as these are encouraging to people teaching in adult literacy programs. They may also inspire other professionals and friends to encourage and facilitate literacy (or any other basic life skill) for the older adult. The fact that a person has fewer years to use a life skill does not and should not make it any less important and fulfilling to that person. In fact, it may be quite the opposite. Similarly, for the literacy tutor, the shortage of years presents a limited time to make a difference.

Participation of older persons in various educational, volunteer, and travel programs is often motivated by a longtime desire to be connected with aspects of the local and larger community, combined with the availability of time and resources. For some, Extended Middle Age provides the window of opportunity to engage the wish list of a lifetime. For others, the window opening is much less expansive, providing limited time and the constraint of limited resources. In this instance, opportunities may be focused on local organizations, such as the church, or on the extended family and friends. Don, with limited resources and a fear of travel, found Extended Middle Age to be a time to assist neighbors, many of whom were elderly, with home maintenance tasks and household chores. Never in all his years had he been so indispensable. Some have been able to combine ample measures of work, leisure, and education throughout adulthood and are continuing that combination into older adulthood, so that fulfillment has been a product of the present throughout adulthood, rather than a hope for the future. In any case, an active adaptive response to Extended Middle Age recognizes both the constraints and the opportunities and weaves a web of fulfillment between the two.

This is a time with opportunities for new beginnings, a time of setting out in new directions, a time of enjoyment, one that capitalizes on the great potential with which this period begins.

A SEASON IN SEARCH OF A PURPOSE

The societal context within which these choices are made is one that gives mixed signals and ascribes uncertain functions to older persons. The role of older adults in our society is ambiguous at best, in part because older adulthood is taken as a whole without the differentiation of periods that allows naming and focusing on the specific tasks at hand. It is also the result of a transition from the clearly defined norms of work and adulthood to a setting that lacks clearly stated expectations. Tom Cole calls it a "season in search of a purpose" (1997, p. 59). The impact of this on Extended Middle Age is exacerbated as various elements of the transition into it may have stripped a person, in whole or part, of power, productivity, influence, income, relationships, structure, goals, and, in some instances, independence.

None of the classic models of older adult behavior offers a satisfactory developmental framework for understanding this "season in search of a purpose." Disengagement theory (Cumming & Henry, 1961) is based on the assumption that a principal and normal process of aging is one where the number and quality of relationships between the individual and society are reduced and eventually severed as older adults deliberately seek isolation via the reduction of social contacts. Concurrently, society participates in the process by freeing the aging individual from social commitments. Although the inevitability of this withdrawal from social interaction by older adults has been questioned on empirical grounds (Aschenbaum & Bengtson, 1994), it describes only part of the aging process, ignoring the other half of the adaptive and re-creative process in which persons in Extended Middle Age disengage from particular relationships and activities and simultaneously re-engage in others, motivated by circumstance and context.

Activity theory assumes that life satisfaction increases with social activity (Havighurst, Cavan, Burgess, & Goldhammer, 1949). Whereas disengagement theorists pointed one toward the rocking chair, activity advocates lead one to the volunteer center or the golf course. Many studies have drawn links between levels of various activities and measures ranging from life satisfaction and successful aging to longevity. Present-day activity proponents remind us that if we don't use our bodies and minds, we will lose their capability. "Use it or lose it," they say. "Better to wear out than to rust out." The thrust toward use or activity, no matter how essential to older adult health and well-being, falls flat when there is no strong purpose to be served by that activity. Use without purpose and meaning is pointless and unmotivating.

Proponents of continuity theory (Atchley, 1983) point to the stability of the self throughout adulthood. This stability of self from adulthood to older adulthood suggests that the main themes of older adulthood are a continuation of the themes and pursuits that have dominated adulthood.

While each of these conceptualizations describes one important facet of the older adult experience, they do not (nor were they intended to) provide a comprehensive framework for envisioning the road ahead. Furthermore, changes in the influence of employment and family have reduced their ability to shape life's purpose as they once did. Now that purpose and meaning are not imposed, one has to choose them. For some, this is a time of eager anticipation. They've been "chompin' at the bit," waiting to get to their own agenda. For others, there is a sense of letdown. Mostly, they had been content in the flow of their work and family years and had no great desire to "fly solo."

Not everyone moves at the same speed or has the same need for structure. One man, three years retired, said he had re-invented who he would be in retirement at least five times. Another, also three years retired, said, "I go to the correctional center to counsel with folks on Thursday evenings, and I have a prayer meeting on Friday morning— and that's all the structure I need for my week." Others might need to get on a more scheduled path or have greater or fewer activities to structure their time.

Discovering the Options

What activities will consume Extended Middle Age? What will be a person's vocation (from the Latin, meaning "calling") for the latter years? What is each to do or to be? In other words, what is the purpose of this time in a person's life? Visions of retirement as a vacation are a far cry from the need to make choices about retirement as vocation. Burton and Doris Kreitlow (1997) call this a "retirement career." A retirement career is what you do with your life in older adulthood. Novelist Gale Godwin (1999) writes, "Something is your vocation if it keeps making more of you" (p. 12).

Most choices at this life stage are concerned to provide a meaningful substitute for paid work or a meaningful supplement to full- or part-time employment. Many find volunteer responsibilities to be worthy work surrogates or supplements, as indicated by the 46 percent of persons aged 65 to 74 who participate in volunteer activities on an average of 3.6 hours per week (Independent Sector, 1999). Other choices at this point in the last third of life include family responsibilities, recreational and travel activities, professional activity, study, or a new career. There is also a default option, "none of the above," when what is chosen is whatever comes along, or when what is chosen is whatever others initiate.

Whether by choice or necessity, some arrive in retirement only to return to the work world. They follow this path either to escape the emptiness and boredom of the days ahead of them or because they like the structure and chance to meet new people that work provides. And some, of course, simply choose to supplement their income. A discount store commercial captures this mind-set when an older greeter declares, "Retirement is for the birds. I'd rather work!" Retirement goals, if they exist, may include a return to employment, although most likely in a less-stressful and often lower-paying job.

Good Choices

Good choices require an identification of the capacities, talents, and interests that are to be used or developed or that indirectly reflect on what will be done with the rest of life. Unless one is able to use abilities for some productive activity, questions of the purpose and value of that person's life, esteem, and value are pervasive. According to Abraham Maslow (1971), life is a process of making choices: Some choices are positive, leading toward some work or calling for the well-being of the community and others. Some choices are regressive, born of fear and vulnerability, moving one defensively toward safety. To be captured entirely by regressive choices is to live in fear of appearing foolish or of losing control as one refuses to give away time, resources, or commitment. Obviously, each person makes choices from a continuum ranging from positive to negative. One's pondering about choices might include asking questions of oneself: To what should I devote these next several years while I still have high energy and a sense of personal well-being? Are there causes, institutions, or civic issues that are important to me that need my skills and talents?

Jimmy Carter quotes a friend as advising, "We worry too much about something to live on—and too little about something to live for" (Carter, 1998, p. 94). What point would there be to a life without goals or purpose, or life in which there is no growth? Good choices lead to increased meaning and purpose in activities, new experiences, relationships, autonomy, and in the ability to continue making choices as the stages of older adulthood unfold.

While not all older persons see themselves as leaders, nearly every person has a valuable and unique contribution to make. Some might call it a legacy, or "making a difference." Everyone needs the space to make a difference—to have the freedom to make choices that have an impact. Not everyone has had that opportunity during years laden with family and work. For example, many persons, especially workers in factories and offices, have had little control in their working lives. Punching a time clock, fitting neatly into a hierarchical structure with little discretion about how to perform tasks, these men and women have had to hold in abeyance many notions of autonomy or control. Now some are highly motivated to seek it. "Retirement is when no one tells you what to do—and you must obey" was one person's definition of the years after work. Once out from under the tyranny of the paycheck there may be a new kind of opportunity to make a difference.

Everyday life is about both physical survival and what it takes to sustain oneself as a human being. After taking care of the survival, maintenance, and development of self and those who count on us, there is still the larger task of what Flacks (1988) calls "history making" or Erikson (1950) calls "generativity." Both focus on making a difference and tending to the survival, maintenance, and development of society. Both are deeply tied to choices that spring from a sense of autonomy joined to a sense of caring.

A SUBSTITUTE FOR WORK

Whatever the choice, a level of intentionality and personal investment is required in the search to replace the benefits that work provided beyond the paycheck. When asked what they valued about their work, a group of young professionals listed 401(k) plans, social interaction, fulfillment, satisfaction, success, knowledge, structure, time away from family, value, status, and identity as valuable outcomes of working. Work structured time—indeed it consumed it. One never needed to schedule a day: the job did it. It gave the worker a sense of productivity, if not accomplishment. In addition, most work presented challenges: the demand to learn new things, face challenges, develop increased competencies, fulfill new requirements, and keep up with constantly advancing technology. There were also collegial relationships and in many cases close friendships. Most jobs were with people and contained an important social dimension, whether welcome or not. Giving up work meant giving up a way of life—a reason for being, an organizer of time, a means of accomplishment, and a source of relationships. These benefits of work, along with income, disappeared with the job, creating a void.

The significance of various aspects of work differ from person to person. Time without purpose may weigh heavy. Time without structure may be chaotic. Time without relationships may be lonely. The positive aspects of older people living longer is lost if their lives lack meaning, purpose, and enjoyment.

The choices, of course, depend on the individual and the context. Some individuals are very intentional about the choices they make. For them, for example, lunch with former colleagues maintains valued relationships. Dividing the day into blocks of time—one set aside for volunteering, one for physical work, and one for reading and chatting with friends—gives it priority and order and rescues it from the confusion of conflicting interests, or the ennui of no interests at all. Others refuse to set up any structure and accept whatever happens, often allowing others to choose for them.

Multiple voices describe retirement in ways that range from the highly active to the very passive. Colleagues and friends may provide models, but, according to Burton and Doris Kreitlow (1997), the key factors that determine how one shapes retirement choices are these: the desire or need to earn income during the retirement years, the need to help other people and develop personal relationships, the need to influence society and improve the well-being of others, the need to maintain some level of autonomy or independence over one's time and schedule, the need for time alone, and the need to be challenged by new experiences and new learning. In their research, the Kreitlows found that "the person who is positively retired is more independent than dependent, more engaged in society than disengaged, more satisfied with retirement than dissatisfied, and freer to make their own choices than to be controlled by others" (p. 12).

What to Do?

In Fisher's (1993) study, most of the activities in which persons engaged, such as handwork or woodworking, had been learned many years earlier and had served as lifetime hobbies. Along with uses of discretionary time for volunteer service, hobbies and interests had been interrupted by more pressing concerns. Many persons are able to revisit a hobby left behind and direct it toward an activity that provides community benefit—Habitat for Humanity, a work camp for junior highs, delivering meals to the homebound. Some choose activities and pursuits they have never tried before. Fortunately, the opportunity of this period allows for both the familiar and the new, the comfortable and the adventurous. The choices are constrained only by circumstance, interest, and imagination.

Some activities were carried forward from work: a professional secretary now worked as a volunteer secretary, and a former teacher volunteered at a nearby private school. Nearly every interviewee spoke of the amount of time currently available that had been absent during the working and child-rearing years. One said, "I think that retirement is doing things better than you had a chance to do . . . at your own pace." A very active woman spoke of this as a time when she was "no longer a slave to my house" and could get out and enjoy other activities. Conversely, several women who had worked outside the home spoke of retirement as the time when they could devote more time to homemaking tasks. One woman who had been a teacher thought of retirement in these terms: "I just wanted to keep house. I had thirty years of working and I wanted to stay home and enjoy myself."

Although many women and men referred to this time as carefree, they also expressed concern. Some were concerned about the adequacy of their financial resources. Others spoke of the state of their own health and the health of their mates, parents, children, and friends. As if to combat impending ill health or disability, many spoke of the need to stay active. Others had a fear of any physical malady the future might bring. One said, "I have a horror of being incapacitated if I live to be 92 as my mother did." Another spoke of singing at a nursing home and seeing the different people there. She said, "You wonder which one you're going to be like. It's rather frightening—I think I'm going to be a very disagreeable old lady!" Nearly all were concerned about the number of years they had left to live. One man said the worst thing about being his age was that he wouldn't be around for the next 50 years. One woman had hoped for an even greater level of continuity with middle age than actually materialized. She anticipated that she and her husband "would maybe travel and do things together . . . but when he retired, he didn't want to travel; he wanted to stay home. So we never did get anyplace."

A particular concern for some persons, particularly women, in Extended Middle Age is the demand to be caregivers for their frail parents. Frail older adults are particularly vulnerable, and about three-quarters of them depend on volunteer caregivers. The community-based frail and dependent population is large (about 8.7 million people age 65 and older in 2002), many live alone, most have modest financial resources, and many depend on help from family—often a daughter—or friends. As noted in a recent report on frail older adults and their caregivers (Johnson & Wiener, 2006),

> long-term care is a women's issue. . . . Daughters account for about 7 of every 10 adult children who help their frail parents and about five of every six who assume primary responsibility for their personal care. . . . [Such caregivers] average 201 hours of help per month, more than the typical full-time job. (pp. vii-viii)

Through this Extended Middle Age, many of the interests and activities of middle age were pursued. In fact, it resembled middle age sans work for those who had worked outside the home. Whatever plans most persons had for retirement were designed for this period. The demands of caregiving, of course, can be extraordinarily disruptive of even the best-laid plans.

Learning Activities

A recent study found that older people are engaged in formal learning in increasing numbers and amounts of time. According to the

National Center for Educational Statistics, the percentage of people in the United States between the ages of 65 and 69 who took at least one adult education class in the previous year increased from 14 percent in 1991 to 25 percent in 1999, and those 70 years of age and above increased from 9 percent in 1991 to 15 percent in 1999 (National Center for Educational Statistics, 2001, Table 359). In 1996, nearly 14 percent of persons age 65 and above participated in courses for personal development and over 2 percent participated in a work-related course (Stowe, 1996). Since participation in educational activities by adults is strongly correlated with their own educational attainment, participation will likely continue to increase as the median level of educational attainment in the older adult population increases.

Howard McClusky (1971) has described the learning needs of older adults as coping, expressive, contributive, influential, and transcendent. Although his projection that older persons possessed learning needs seemed well ahead of its time, his description takes into account both the diversity of the population and their wide variety of needs to survive through improved work-related or personal management skills; to increase enrichment through courses in arts and crafts, the humanities, or travel; to improve well-being; to make a difference; and to affirm oneself in the larger scheme of things.

Learning opportunities often accessed by those in Extended Middle Age include national organizations such as Institutes for Learning in Retirement, noncredit programs sponsored by individual colleges and universities designed for older learners; Elderhostel, a program involving 300,000 persons over 50 in a variety of travel and enrichment opportunities in the United States and abroad; OASIS (Older Adult Service and Information Systems), a program based in 30 shopping centers serving 300,000 older persons; SeniorNet, a computer network with over 100 centers where older persons are taught computer use; and Shepherd's Centers, a community service and educational organization located at churches and synagogues (Manheimer, Snodgrass, & Moskow-McKenzie, 1995). In many areas, colleges and universities offer tuition-free auditing privileges. Most senior centers respond to educational needs and interests through educational programs, as do other institutions, such as churches, libraries, community colleges, and businesses. Self-directed learning activities have been aided by the use of computers; in 2000, 28 percent of persons 65 years of age had home computers and 13 percent had use of the Internet at home

(U.S. Census Bureau, 2000b). And, of course, the plethora of educational institutions and programs designed for adults in general are available and used by older persons as well.

Although participation in learning activities is rewarded by the acquisition of new knowledge, skills, and interests as well as new experiences, the greatest benefit may come from the opportunities they present for socialization (Fisher, 1986). The practice of participation in learning activities begun in Extended Middle Age is frequently continued at varying levels in available venues through the subsequent periods of older adulthood.

Professionals who serve as teachers or mentors with older students can develop a supportive learning climate, clarify the structure and organization of the material to be learned, encourage older adult learners to persist in their learning, allow for individual pacing of instruction, and strengthen the connection between current and new information (Fisher, 1998, p. 32). Whether the best setting for older adult learning occurs in an age-integrated or age-segregated environment often depends on the educational background and comfort level of the learner as well as the subject area to be taught.

RELATIONSHIPS AND SOLITUDE

The challenges of Extended Middle Age include freedom—finding one's new voice, new self, and meaning—making sense of a time of life with no clear socially given meaning. These two topics have been dealt with extensively in this chapter. There are also two other topics to consider: relationships and solitude, and balancing gains and losses.

Choices that provide worth and affirm purpose are not made in a vacuum or in isolation. The restructuring of purpose is often accompanied by the restructuring of relationships: workplace colleagues are no longer available, and neighbors and friends relocate. On the other hand, many peers are also exploring new relationships for similar reasons. Common interests or similar causes provide important opportunities to make new friends. Studies of what influences older adults to participate in learning activities and other events reveal that socialization is one of the most important motivators. Relationships are an important by-product of activities in the older adult world.

In the years of work and family, friends seem to have just happened. Jobs, church, neighborhoods, clubs—all provided opportunities for acquaintances and friends. As that supply tends to dwindle over time, it may provoke little notice, but it creates a situation that demands attention. In older adulthood, circumstances change and making friends becomes a more deliberate activity. The need to be more intentional in making friends is more characteristic of males than females, whose circles of friends and networks of support tend to be broader and more inclusive. For the person who is shy, the actions needed to make friends may involve a certain level of discomfort. But, generally, older adults who have friends are persons who have engaged actively and consistently in the business of making friends and creating strong relationships.

In this period, even for the outgoing person, the diminishing parade of passing family and friends becomes noticeable. But beginning with Extended Middle Age, older adults turn to close friends for emotional support as well as satisfying relationships. This will intensify in later periods. Choosing an approach to living that emphasizes making friends is a critical first step in warding off potential aloneness and loneliness in later years. One Extended Middle Age man has developed a "lunch list." When potential friends casually remark, "Let's get together," he adds the name to the list. Each week he schedules lunch with a new name from the list. Selecting someone with whom to maintain a conversation of mutual interest during a meal is integral to his process of friend-making and friend-keeping.

William Thomas (2004) describes the three plagues of older adulthood as loneliness, helplessness, and boredom. A cadre of persons with whom one engages in continuing and active relationships—family members, friends, fellow members of religious and other organizations, colleagues, and former colleagues—goes a long way toward fending off these plagues.

The presence of friends during the early years of retirement often eases the burden on husbands and wives who may suddenly be cast in the role of "only friends" of each other. This 24-hour togetherness, often for the first time in a marriage, may impose unexpected strains. However, Weiss (2005, p. 185) concludes from his extensive research that "[m]ost couples, including those who are initially apprehensive about getting in each other's way, wind up pleased by the increase in their time together." This does not, of course, preclude time alone.

Grandchildren may be a source of companionship, at least for some. The central media-driven image of modern American grandparenting portrays the relationship between grandparent and grandchild in terms of equality, love, affection, and friendship. For many retirees a trip to visit the grandchildren is one of the highlights of the year. Companion grandparenting is not for everyone, however, as new caregiving demands can make the relationship one of being a parent all over again—and often without nine months to plan for it (Dressel, 1996, p. 80).

An increasing number of grandparents, however, find themselves with responsibility as primary caregivers, guardians, or surrogate parents to their own grandchildren. In 2000, 21 percent of those taking care of their grandchildren were aged 60 to 69. Although grandparents serving as surrogate parents represent all socioeconomic and ethnic groups, they are more likely to be black, Hispanic, or Native American than non-Hispanic white or Asian, and more likely to be poorer than in a parent-maintained family (Simmons & Dye, 2003, p. 8). In some instances, being cast in the role of surrogate parents comes as an unanticipated intrusion into the latter years and an interruption of the plans made for this time. In other situations, more likely in African-American families as well as some other ethnic traditions, a grandmother parenting her grandchildren, as well as assorted other young family members, casts her in a familiar and not unexpected role. Indeed, she may have been reared by her own grandmother and may see this as the role that her cultural tradition defines for her, or, on the other hand, she may have become sufficiently acculturated by the dominant culture to expect her children to care for their own offspring.

ALONENESS AND INDEPENDENCE

The emphasis on relationships needs to be juxtaposed with the need for aloneness and independence. If friendship is built on compromise and consensus, one needs also to have a time for autonomy, where one's sense of self-control and self-esteem make time alone a productive source of goodwill and pride. Time alone may be time to confront fears and self-doubts. Time alone may be time to develop a richer inner life or to embark on or continue a spiritual journey. A common claim, "I've never been busier than I am now," may mask an inability to deal with the challenges and opportunities of aloneness and solitude.

One important aspect of Extended Middle Age is the exploration of the bounds of freedom and autonomy. Not many will push the bounds of socially acceptable behavior, but questions of aloneness or togetherness for couples and questions of being "in town" or "on the road" for family and friends are ways the bounds of freedom are tested. Crucial tests often revolve around decision making involving individual and family concerns where family members do not feel they have been adequately consulted. Individual comforts and patterns of decision making will determine just where these boundaries will be drawn in Extended Middle Age.

BALANCING GAINS AND LOSSES

As the pattern of this period unfolds, it clearly resembles a balancing act, recognizing the important losses incurred and the choices that must be made to compensate for them, and even to turn them into gains. The loss that overshadows this period is usually that of employment in which the physical, economic, social, and psychological perquisites of work fade away and are replaced with involvement in causes and activities that provide for survival, self-enrichment, and/or the common good. The gradual loss of friends and colleagues is supplanted by gaining new friends and acquaintances who share similar interests. And the loss of dominant time-structuring pursuits, such as a full-time, paid job, opens into the freedom to exercise greater control over one's time through the choices made.

Never will the need to make meaningful choices about life's purpose be absent, and it will be accompanied by the challenge to engage in fulfilling relationships, and to address issues of autonomy, control, and loss. The environment in which persons live will surround them with changes requiring continued adaptation to the new circumstances. Current values in every cultural tradition seem to be forgetful of "the old ways."

This period in which middle age is continued into older adulthood presents the fewest constraints—one might say imposes the fewest losses—and therefore eases people into the process however gently. It also occurs at a time when persons are best equipped to deal with it by virtue of the decisions they make plus the availability of comparatively good health and financial resources. For this reason, during Extended Middle Age a person is least likely to need the services of a professional.

This period for most is one of stretching middle age as far as possible, and of anticipating the transitions and stable periods to come. Thinking ahead about what life is for in the face of subsequent losses and about where to find friendship and support may assist the future periods to be times of fulfillment, achievement, and growth. Yet, as Mary Pipher (1999) notes, "The saddest thing about old age isn't loss but the failure to grow from experiences" (p. 192). It is by helping members of the Extended Middle Age group analyze and learn from their experience as newly minted older adults that professionals and family members may provide invaluable assistance and support and help them anticipate future tasks and encourage careful planning.

THE ROLE OF THE HELPING PROFESSIONS

Some people will need help negotiating a satisfying Extended Middle Age. Most will not find it easy to connect with people in the helping professions who are experts in this part of the journey of life. Some will, with varying degrees of success, seek counseling for "adjustment disorders." Some will find life coaches who are experts in helping people negotiate many aspects of Extended Middle Age. There are a few of these, but only a few. Some will find help in educational activities specifically geared to this time of life. The number of these is growing.

When the challenges of the whole of the last third of the journey of life become better understood and more widely discussed it will be more likely that people who need and seek help will find competent guides.

Chapter 4

The Early Transition

For six years after they both retired, Manny and Ed lived rich, purposeful lives. Their days were filled with volunteering—Ed taught woodworking at the Boys and Girls Club, Manny did graphic design for nonprofits,
and together they engaged the yearly rhythms of home and hearth,
family and friends. One June morning, just as he was leaving for the
Boys and Girls Club, Ed experienced numbness in the left side of his
body. His vision got blurry and his head hurt terribly. When he tried to
tell Manny what was wrong he had problems speaking. She called 911
and got him to the emergency room. In spite of prompt medical care,
the stroke did damage that physical therapy couldn't completely cure.
Ed was alive and quite well, but forever changed. The great love of his
volunteer life, teaching woodworking, was ended. This marked a turn-
ing point in Manny's and Ed's lives.

Ed's identity had been deeply—and healthily—tied up in his volunteer work and his life with Manny. He and Manny were longtime
friends, parents of three children, and companions who now were enjoying a new depth of conversation, parallel volunteer projects that
enriched their lives, a deep sense of caring and new ways to express
it, interdependence, and good sexual intimacy (Moss & Schwebel,
1993). So much had now to be renegotiated as the result of his illness.
It was a dark journey that only came out into a new light after almost a
year of struggle.

The events that comprise the Early Transition—always life changing, often involuntary—are characterized both by their seriousness
and by their uncertainty. On the way to the hospital, Manny knew in-
stinctively that things would not soon return to normal, if ever. But
exactly where they would lead was uncertain as well. More than one

A Journey Called Aging: Challenges and Opportunities in Older Adulthood
© 2007 by The Haworth Press, Taylor & Francis Group. All rights reserved.
doi:10.1300/5915_05

person has compared the beginning of the Early Transition with the entry to a tunnel—the light diminished, the path constrained by walls of circumstance, the exit obscured, life and light on the other side not visible from the entry. Nor is there information at the beginning just how long the tunnel or the transition will last.

Many introductions to the Early Transition begin with an ambulance ride, but not all. Others begin with shortness of breath, not feeling up to par, a fall, a routine visit to the doctor that reveals an unexpected and potentially serious finding, or the diagnosis of a terminal condition. No abstraction, such as "illness," can lessen the trauma.

The intrusion of a serious physical health problem brings immediate consequences. Activities and schedules are changed to accommodate the limitations imposed by the malady as well as the treatment regimen. Other family members and friends become involved as caregivers. Nurses, therapists, and others providing assistance become regular home visitors. Schedules are built around appointments and interactions with a broad range of health care professionals. Work, volunteer, and leisure activities are suspended; social activities may be impossible, except for brief visits by a few close friends. And the "crisis mode" that was created by the initial event settles into a routine as the regimen of care and therapy continues.

Many of the questions that such an event imposes boil down to these: How long? How long in the hospital? When will treatment be completed? How much time until recovery is complete? These questions often are surrogates for others: Will therapy or treatment be successful? Is recovery possible, even likely? As one husband stated when his wife was unexpectedly diagnosed with cancer, "This cloud will always hang over us." The future is obscured by unknowns. Little is clear except the pervading uncertainty. Taking "one day at a time" seems like a long-range plan.

An event of such magnitude puts an end to Extended Middle Age. The event may be the death of a spouse, an illness from which one never fully recovers, a one-sided divorce, or the growing realization that one needs a safer, less demanding, more supportive environment in which to live. The presence of change and need for accommodation, uncertainty about the present and future, and the inability to sustain a middle-age lifestyle are indicators of the Early Transition. Whether its inception is voluntary or involuntary, the Early Transition cuts across

Extended Middle Age and effectively terminates that Extended Middle Age lifestyle.

This chapter encourages all who accompany persons during these events to understand the transitional process—one in which grieving the passing of persons, possessions, health, and even a lifestyle, is a natural as well as a necessary component. Those who serve this population, whether as professionals or loving family members and friends, are encouraged to offer support for the long haul and cautioned not to impose inappropriate expectations on those who require time and energy for grieving loss, addressing change, adapting to a new way of life, and possibly discovering a new reason for living.

VOLUNTARY AND INVOLUNTARY APPROACHES

In its most graphic (and often most devastating) form, the events of the transition interrupt the flow of the lives of the persons directly involved. But family, friends, and even associated professionals are not left untouched. In this form, persons are caught up in the transition involuntarily—it comes to them. Among the interviewees in Fisher's (1993) study, it was the Early Transition that, more than anything else, encompassed the decisive events that changed the dynamics of life. A veritable line in the sand, after which nothing is the same— Ed's stroke, the onset of life-altering illness, the death of a spouse, the need to relocate, followed closely by the direct consequence of each event. These include a range of adjustments required by the new situation as well as the challenge to maintain a sense of control and direction in the midst of new circumstances and new dependencies.

In a less dramatic but equally pivotal fashion, others enter this transition voluntarily, as a matter of choice. Although prompted by circumstances and a sense of their own mortality, people elect to make significant lifestyle changes that often include downsizing their residence and possessions, giving up certain responsibilities and activities, and focusing more directly on the years ahead. The choices that lead one to initiate this transition may center on health: a shortness of breath that occurs occasionally—a reminder that it was shortness of breath that preceded a father's fatal heart attack—or the awareness that one has already lived longer than either parents or siblings, or that one's stamina and decision-making ability are no longer what they once were. The choices may be prompted by concern for one's own emotional or mental equilibrium, or a feeling of being overwhelmed by present obligations or circumstances, or the transitions being experienced by peers along the journey of older adulthood.

Whether voluntary or involuntary, this transition comes with a sense of diminishment: the abundant and sometimes carefree opportunities of Extended Middle Age, the options of work and leisure inherent in that time, are curtailed. The expansiveness of Extended Middle Age gives way to contraction and even the vision of potential disintegration.

In many respects, the Early Transition, no respecter of persons, is the great leveler of older adulthood. Descriptions of Extended Middle Age have focused on a number of key factors: financial resources, use of discretionary time, the need or desire for employment, professional commitments, family linkages, and others. No matter whether Extended Middle Age is consumed by the interesting use of leisure or by continued employment out of necessity, the Early Transition comes unabated. Neither social class, financial resources, ethnicity, nor gender excuse one. Certainly there are linkages between socioeconomic status and health and health care; nevertheless, for each individual, partnership, and family network, there come those events that terminate whatever agenda Extended Middle Age held and introduce another lifestyle.

Demographic Landmarks

The difference between the Early Transition at 70 and the Early Transition at 80 is enormous for any one given individual. At 80, one may be more likely to admit that the Early Transition is more or less "on time." Not so at age 70, or for the great many of all ages for whom it comes much too soon.

Yet, locating the events of the Early Transition at a particular age poses several problems. First, these events do not occur at the same time for every individual. For some, this transition may occur earlier in older adulthood (in their sixties, for example) or later (in their early eighties). Second, many of the events that are pivotal to the transition are cumulative. Health may begin to deteriorate decades earlier and finally impose significant changes on lifestyle at this transitional point. Nevertheless, demographic indicators describing the incidence of events of the Early Transition point to changes that occur most frequently in the seventies.

With regard to the death of a spouse, the probability of dying increases dramatically from the years between 65 and 70 to the years between 75 and 80. A person is more than twice as likely to die between the years of 75 and 80 (probability = .20557) than between the years 65 and 70 (probability = .09217) (U.S. Department of Health and Human Services, 2002, Table 3). Consequently, 9 percent of men between the ages of 65 and 74 are widowed, whereas 18 percent between the ages of 75 and 84 are widowed. Similarly, 31 percent of women between the ages of 65 and 74 are widowed, and 55 percent between the ages of 75 and 84 are widowed (*Older Americans 2000: Key Indicators of Well-Being*, 2000, Appendix A, Indicator 3).

Another consequence of increased mortality is a change in the male-female ratio. In the 65 to 74 age category, there are 83 males for every 100 females in the population. In the 75 to 84 age category, the number drops to 67 males for every 100 females, clearly an indicator of changes brought about by death during this time period (U.S. Census Bureau, 2003c).

Furthermore, the percentage of those living with their spouses diminishes significantly with age. Most of those who are left are women: over 50 percent of women of age 75 or older live alone, compared with 30 percent of women of age 65 to 74. This compares with 23 percent of men age 75 or older and 13 percent of men age 65 to 74 who live alone (*Older Americans 2000: Key Indicators of Well-Being*, 2000, Appendix A, Indicator 3). Illness begins to increase, as measured by the increase in health care expenditures: health care expenditures increase by 50 percent on average between 65 and 75 years of age, according to a Medicare Current Beneficiary Survey (*Older Americans 2000: Key Indicators of Well-Being*, 2000, Indicator 5). Men and women are three times as likely to suffer moderate or severe memory impairment at age 75 than at age 65 (*Older Americans 2000: Key Indicators of Well-Being*, 2000, Indicator 15). The percentage of persons of all races who report having good or excellent health declines from the age group 65 to 74 to the age group 75 to 84 (*Older Americans 2000: Key Indicators of Well-Being*, 2000, Indicator 17).

One may view these data describing changes that occur in the seventies as a product of the data collection system that uses the mid-seventies simply as a point in chronological time to differentiate an earlier age (65-74) from a later one (75-84). One may also view these data as a summary of human experience during these years. In either event, they record significant changes in mortality, illness, and related problems when the early years of older adulthood are compared with the decade following, anchoring most of these changes in the seventies. These data describe the Early Transition, that process of concluding middle age and moving into an Older Adult Lifestyle. Precisely when (at what age) it happens for any individual is not predictable. Ultimately statistics are only helpful for large numbers, never when $n = 1$.

BETWIXT AND BETWEEN

Admittedly some transitions are more life changing than others. Most older adults have first-hand experience with transitions. They have lived through adolescence, first job, marriage, first baby, and other events of adulthood. Furthermore, they have likely watched and participated vicariously as their children and grandchildren maneuver these same passages.

Anthropologists and ethnographers studying complex patterns of major life transition use the term *liminal,* from the Latin *limen,* meaning "threshold." For example, studies of the initiation of adolescents into adulthood among traditional peoples in various cultures describe a series of ordeals and rituals—sometimes taking months or even a year—through which they shed their childhood and emerge as adults ready to take up their work in the community. In this process there is a "betwixt and between" phase between childhood and adulthood, where the child is not a child any longer, but not yet an adult. This is the liminal or threshold phase (Trubshaw, 1995). The "betwixt and between" phase of the Early Transition is qualitatively different and potentially more significant and tumultuous than any of life's previous transitions that involved the simple, anticipated passages occurring earlier in adulthood. The Early Transition from one state to another is, in degrees of intensity, liminal. A threshold must be crossed. The experience may be profoundly upsetting. The person who passes through the transition will emerge on the other side having been cut loose from previously satisfactory answers to the defining questions "Who am I? What do I do? With whom do I do it?" The one crossing the threshold may feel disoriented, without clear guiding markers, with a diminished sense of self or identity, or lacking compelling reason to continue.

> Sally and Jim have lived in their dream home with a broad view of the lake—a home they designed and built—for over ten years. Recently topics such as maintenance and upkeep, condos, and dealing with decades of accumulated possessions have infiltrated their conversation. But the discussions are laced with much equivocation. One day condos look like a promising alternative. The next day the conversation explores hiring a service to maintain their property. They have begun the process of downsizing by giving away a few unused furnishings. No overt factors are forcing a decision now, but they are convinced a decision should be made. Between conversations over several months there is much anguish, for both know there is no return from the decision once made. Will a decision to stay simply postpone the inevitable decision to relocate? And if now is not the right time, when?

Even when the change is voluntary, this is the nature of the liminal—one foot standing in the before, the other searching for solid footing in the after. In it, a person must redefine some basic life categories, and in so doing let go of earlier ones. New answers await to be formulated, a new identity to be forged and formed. Fundamental questions about purpose and relationships seek new answers appropriate to a new situation.

Looking Ahead

People look ahead to this time with a sense of uneasiness, apprehension, even dread. What will happen if Extended Middle Age ends in death for one partner or friend? Can one get along without the other? Can one care for the other through long-term illness or disability? What will happen if the strengths that have carried and sustained, happily, through Extended Middle Age erode, or the family home must be given up? What will happen when the lifestyle formerly enjoyed cannot be continued? What if? When? How? The questions are real. To varying degrees this uncertainty becomes a source of anticipation if not worry.

There may be early anticipations of loss in an illness or a setback—a cold that drags on for the whole winter, an eye operation, a lump the doctor found on a recent examination, joints that demand increasing medical attention, a simple recovery interrupted by a massive infection, or incidents of lessened mental capacity. Perhaps the illness or death of a friend or sibling triggers worry. It may be simply a shadow that darkens the mind during moments of quiet. Call it being morbid, or just realistic. In either case, it prompts wondering and threatens disintegration. It requires thinking ahead, planning ahead.

Teilhard de Chardin (1960) speaks of the seeds of diminishment and loss people carry with themselves in this way:

> Other [intruders] were lying in wait for us later on and appeared as suddenly and brutally as an accident, or as stealthily as an illness. All of us one day or another will come to realize, if we have not already done so, that one of these processes of disorganization has installed itself at the very heart of our lives. Sometimes it is the cells of the body that rebel or become diseased; at other times the very elements of our personality seem to be in conflict or to run amok. And then we impotently stand by and watch collapse, rebellion and inner tyranny, and no friendly influence can come to our help. (pp. 53-54)

Although earlier in life there is the awareness that one's days are numbered, now the anticipation of a loss or major decline is both real and uncertain. One caregiver said, "We are alive and we are together. That beats the alternatives." When a long future stretches out ahead, the losses have a different character than when the road ahead seems shorter. A friend described a communication with his son:

> When his screenwriter son turned 50, he wrote his dad: "I find myself ruminating about what legacy, if any, I will leave as a screenwriter. These thoughts inspire me to drink coffee, rush out to my office and type away, in hopes of writing that one truly excellent script before some impolite fellow with a scythe intervenes." The screenwriter's father replied, "At fifty you've begun to think about Death. The preoccupation tends to grow, though we seldom talk about it, and at 80+ it brings its knitting and sits by the fire. But it is not the actual lightning strike that bothers so much as the uncertainty."

NAMING THE REALITIES

As the exploration of this Early Transition unfolds, there emerges the need to name some of the realities of this difficult time. The basic concept of life as a weaving of transition and stable times is enriched by developing a vocabulary that explores in more detail the process of life-changing transitions. No one comes through the Early Transition unscathed by life's losses. The human experience is that those who have gone through transitions have balanced gains and losses. They have gained some specific life skills in the process to be useful in future transitions.

Mourning

With losses comes grief. With grief comes mourning. When it is a spouse, a loved friend, a partner, a close member of an extended family network, or a companion of many years who has died, there is an expectation that a person will mourn, at least for a period of time. But sometimes help goes awry. Some will try to help a person put a loss behind too quickly. Adult children will clean out closets "so Dad won't have to always be thinking about Mom." As well-intentioned as this approach may be, it misses the role of time in getting from the brokenness of the loss to a sense of reconnecting with the one who died. Or a widow's group will have a rule (this is a true story) that there can't be any unhappiness shared in their meetings, completely missing the need to grieve in active engagement with other mourners. Or well-meaning friends may continue to treat the person as she always was, without giving space and encouragement for the emergence of a new sense of self in recognition of a new status.

Where the loss is different—other than the death of a spouse—a network even of good, smart, well-intentioned friends may have trouble coping. Professionals and others may be tempted to disregard other sources of deep pain and loss. The loss of a partner is public and explicit. But there are other losses that come with their own brands of devastation. How does one relate to a person who is grieving the loss of good health, for example, if a person is now in a wheelchair? How does one deal with the grief and mourning of a person who has lost access to his workshop or studio or even a lifelong hobby because he was forced to relocate into smaller quarters? How does one support the mourning of a person whose partner of 35 years has walked out the door? Or how does one relate to a couple who are voluntarily downsizing their lives, giving up an Extended Middle Age filled with travel, adventure, and excitement, and remembering with joy and sadness what has been but will never be again? The same rules apply: with loss comes grief; with grief comes mourning. And mourning requires time, a context for sharing the grief, and support for the gradual emergence of a new person (Hagman, 2001).

Joan Didion (2005) describes her experience of grief:

> Grief turns out to be a place none of us know until we reach it. . . . We imagine that the moment to most severely test us will be the funeral, after which this hypothetical healing will take place. . . . We have no way of knowing that the funeral itself will be anodyne, a kind of narcotic regression in which we are wrapped in the care of others and the gravity and meaning of the occasion. Nor can we know ahead of the fact (and here lies the heart of the difference between grief as we imagine it and grief as it is) the unending absence that follows, the void, the very opposite of meaning, the relentless succession of moments during which we will confront the experience of meaninglessness itself. (pp. 188-189)

Not all agree on the nature of grieving, or the outcome of mourning. For some, it is the restoration of a psychic equilibrium, a return to the health of that time before the loss occurred, and it occurs for the most part in private. Others see mourning as transformational rather than merely restorative, as occurring with the support and dialogue of friends rather than in private, and as looking forward rather than back. In this view, one goal of mourning is to "reconnect," but in a new way, with what has been lost rather than simply "getting over it." In this latter view, the mourning process is highly individualized, anticipating the development of a new creation. It is not susceptible to a standardized timetable, and requires both sensitivity and support from professionals and friends (Hagman, 2001).

Given a transformational approach to loss and change, it may not be possible to relate to a person as that person used to be. She or he is a new person (or won't survive), and professionals and friends need to begin a long process, with the individual, of discovery of this new person. Similar responses of time, support, and openness to newness are essential ingredients of the mourning process, whatever the loss. One can only hope that those in the Early Transition will receive the support and find the strength to overcome a whole variety of significant, life-changing losses. The reality is encouraging. Many do.

The Dynamics of Transitions

When one recalls the experience of significant transitions earlier in life, such as leaving home in young adulthood, it becomes clear that the transition began with the loss of safety, security, Mom's meals, friends and neighborhood, a relationship with parents, and a home. But to build an adult life, these had to be left behind in the process of finding a job, friends, a place to live, a new way of being a person.

At some point, the gains began to outweigh the losses. After a successful transition into the adult world, a person can return home as an independent adult—perhaps with a spouse or significant other—and successfully negotiate a new way of relating with parents, friends, family, and neighborhood. Home and parents are viewed in new ways; the adolescent turned adult has a new view of home, parents, and self, opening a new chapter in the life story.

The process of moving through loss into gain happens in the life transition of retiring. For example, a woman dreams, saves, plans, announces her decision, and signs the papers. After the glow wears off and she's had that around-the-world trip (literally or figuratively), she gets into a funk (Atchley, 1976). She is now moving into the heart of the transition. And when she finally gets through it, she has found, perhaps, a sense of purpose as a volunteer at the nature center and a sense of avocation as a sculptor that is new and energizing. She owns the losses without dwelling on them; she puts the bad days of the transition behind her, and she makes the most of the gains of her new life even as she reaches back into her work past to find the skills that she needs to be effective today. The same basic pattern—losses followed by gain—will happen in Early Transition, although the stakes may be higher and the road longer than previously experienced.

Bridges (1980) captures the transitional process in three phases: "Endings," "The Neutral Zone," and "The New Beginning." In the first phase, the person is cut off, either willingly or unwillingly, from familiar activities, relationships, setting, or important roles and undergoes a symbolic death experience. The ending process includes separation as a conscious act as well as a reconceptualization of one's identity given the new circumstances. The Neutral Zone is a time of separation, a gap between the old and the new. The emptiness that fills this time is seen as a positive element, one where both energy and perspective receive regeneration, and where the emptiness may be filled with something new. Following the letting go of separation comes the opportunity to begin anew. Bridges cautions against using this model as a simple coping manual and instead encourages its use as a way of engendering personal transformation.

CONSEQUENCE OF AN ILLNESS

A graphic depiction of the Early Transition brought about by illness might show it as an octopus, with tentacles extending in all directions. Instead of a single, discrete event, it results in side effects and consequences that impact a great many areas of life, raise issues that may not have not been the subject of serious consideration heretofore, and involve others in their resolution.

Introduction to Care Resources

Hospital discharges are often contingent upon the presumed availability of sufficient care at home or access to a rehabilitation or extended care facility. Persons who have never considered these needs and options are often stirred into making decisions of significant import and choosing among competing options with little preparation in a brief time frame. This usually prompts a quick review of health and extended care insurance and Medicare benefits. Although the prevailing hope is that the need for any care is temporary, it is also unexpected, and decision makers are frequently unaware both of the care options and of the benefits available to them.

Persons without the necessary insurance benefits or financial resources may become involved in the application process for Medicaid and, at the same time, are limited in their options to facilities that will accept Medicaid patients. Another responsibility befalling both resource-rich and resource-poor persons is organizing available family members and close friends into a caregiving network in order to make possible the return home for recuperation.

Introduction to Caregiving

Spouses, partners, and friends are often cast into new and unfamiliar roles as caregivers. The job description will differ, depending on the illness and the person's particular level of functioning. Personal care and hygiene, travel to appointments for medical care and treatment, food preparation, housekeeping, laundry, shopping, and financial affairs may all be included. The list is notable both for the widespread nature of the responsibilities and for the unpreparedness that the caregiver may experience in performing any of these tasks. Husbands, stereotypically, may be unprepared to undertake food preparation, housekeeping, and laundry chores. Wives, again stereotypically, may be unprepared to assume home management or financial management responsibilities. The caregiver is faced both with the presence of an immediate responsibility and with the need to develop proficiency without preparation time. Furthermore, the person receiving care may be unable to coach or mentor the caregiver in the performance of these tasks.

Caregivers, often unpaid family members or friends, in addition to the care of the person who is ill, must maintain their own health and strength. This may mean the identification of others to assist with short-term care, or of a facility or program to provide "respite care," care designed to allow the primary caregiver a "respite" from caregiving responsibilities. Frequent findings from research describing difficulties caregivers face list a paucity of information about how to perform many caregiving (especially medical) tasks and where to learn about resources available to caregivers.

Traditionally, spouses and daughters have been cast into caregiving roles. However, the demographics of caregiving is changing: the prevalence of women in positions of employment outside the home limits their availability to assume this role. The spouse whose employment is necessary to provide supplementary health insurance may be torn between being a personal caregiver and an insurance provider. Declining birthrates among segments of the population will result in fewer children available to care for their aging parents (Johnson, 2000). The mobility that separates family members by geography results in the unavailability of children to be caregivers for their parents. One consequence of these changing demographics is the increased likelihood that nonfamily members will need to be employed in various caregiving roles, ranging from care manager to home health aide, particularly where there are adequate financial resources.

Mental Health Issues

The tension and uncertainty inherent in the events of the Early Transition combined with new responsibilities on the part of caregivers seem uniquely designed to enhance stress and increase strain, often resulting in challenges to coping. This is particularly true when the person suffering the illness must receive care outside the home for an extended period of time. Many have confessed their great sense of guilt that comes from visiting a loved one in a nursing home. But transferring a person from a rehabilitation facility to the person's residence also brings an increased strain to caregiving. Both a disabled person and that person's caregiver may experience feelings of inadequacy, insecurity, or frustration. Furthermore, these feelings on the part of the patient may be exacerbated by required medications or by the interaction of separate medicines, complicating an already complex treatment plan.

Hurdles Faced by Same-Sex Couples

Laws governing marriage in most states together with traditions that begin with promises to care "for better, for worse, in sickness and in health" give married couples the legal responsibility to make joint decisions regarding care. Furthermore, public benefits from social service agencies for which one marriage partner qualifies usually apply to the other partner as well. However, since same-sex partners are not legally married in most states, benefits that accrue to married couples because one of them is eligible may not be available to both partners in a same-sex relationship. Should nursing-home care be required, other obstacles appear: married persons have a legal right to live in the same room; unmarried couples do not.

In addition, same-sex couples must use legal means to provide each other with medical and legal powers of attorney and to write wills that specifically name each other as beneficiary.

Loss of Driving Privileges

An illness or accident that introduces an older person to the Early Transition often reduces a person's ability to drive an automobile. One consequence of a broken limb or a stroke or heart attack may be the temporary but immediate loss of driving privileges. A loss occurring to the principal driver in the household could result in a complete inability to shop, access health care services, or attend social gatherings. Public transportation may not be available or may not be user-friendly or convenient. Hiring transportation or depending on friends and family to provide it imposes an additional stress and burden on persons faced with mounting obstacles.

Radical Change in Social Activities

Illness and its aftermath impose dramatic changes in one's social life. The ability to visit and be visited and to interact with others is often severely limited with respect to mobility and energy. An older gentleman recuperating from hospitalization lamented the fact that his friends were reluctant to visit him at a nursing home. These limitations require careful and thoughtful planning in order for a person not to be cut off from family and friends.

Holiday festivities and the celebrations of family rituals may present particular challenges where traditions conflict with the circumstances brought about by illness or disability. Recognizing the impossibility of simply repeating past events may lead to the establishment of realistic expectations, critical to avoiding disappointment.

Financial Drain

The regimen of health care that surrounds the victim of serious illness or accident rarely provides occasion to stop to assess costs or measure assets, including insurance. Insurance policies of various sorts plus Medicare may provide a solid coverage for most care and treatment for those covered. However, the cost of items that for one reason or another are not included may quickly become unaffordable, adding stress to an already stressful situation. For example, although Medicare will cover a needed 100 days in a skilled nursing facility, it will not cover personal or custodial care (such as assistance in walking, getting in and out of bed, eating, dressing, bathing, and taking medicine), if that is what is needed. People who have unrealistic expectations of what Medicare will cover are likely to be seriously stressed when they encounter the reality.

Such a situation may lead to several outcomes. Some older adults have been led to continue paid employment in order to pay for medical care, thereby postponing the leisure phase of their retirement. Others who have retired from paid employment have chosen to return. Medical bills have led those without assets to apply for Medicaid and others to declare bankruptcy. And still others have declined to acquire medical care because they could not afford it.

A Harbinger?

One aspect of the uncertainty associated with the Early Transition is in knowing when it is complete, short of death. The fear of recurrence elevates each instance of "not feeling well" to feelings of alarm. Such fears lead to preoccupation with bodily concerns, where small aches heretofore unnoticed assume a greater place and evoke concerns lest they be harbingers of more serious things to come.

An event as discrete as a serious bone fracture or the discovery of an unexpected disease pervades virtually all of one's life. It raises obstacles and issues heretofore unconsidered and presents challenges that further complicate recovery from the event itself. As a result, it is not only the event that ushers in the Early Transition but the surrounding impact of innumerable consequences that force a change in lifestyle terminating Extended Middle Age.

DEATH AND LOSS IN LATER LIFE

Beyond illness, the most basic loss, that which defines all others, is death. All humans are mortal. "Little deaths"—losses, hurts, and diminishments—are part of the fabric of life. Qualitatively, though, loss is different in later life. From midlife when one begins to count time to death instead of time from birth, death casts a shadow that brings into increasingly sharp relief the one-way nature of the human journey.

At the end of *The Shadow Box* (Christofer, 1977), the characters speak in a kind of chorus:

> And then you think, someone should have said it sooner.
> Someone should have said it a long time ago.
> Someone should have said, this living . . .
> . . . this life . . .
> . . . this lifetime . . .
> It doesn't last forever.
> A few days, a few minutes . . . that's all.
> It has an end.
> This face.
> These hands.
> This word.
> It doesn't last forever.
> This air.
> This light.
> This earth.
> These things you love.
> These children.
> This smile.
> This pain.
> It doesn't last forever.
> It was never supposed to last forever. (pp. 85-86)

The insight that it doesn't last forever and was never supposed to last forever is not won without cost. But the insight can be life-giving. To embrace this movement from the unthinkable to the unavoidable is to gain a stronger ability to accept and tolerate conflict and ambivalence. This insight is not something to be avoided; rather it is something to be struggled for. "If [age] is a long defeat it is also a victory, meaningful for the initiates of time, if not for those who have come less far" (Scott-Maxwell, 1968, p. 5).

A dimension of the qualitative difference of loss in older adulthood is a certainty that one's life has taken paths that cannot be retraced. A glaucoma specialist responded to a question about how older adults typically deal with the onset of blindness. "Mostly they are quite stoical. They tell me, 'That's the way it is, I guess.' And then they often add, 'I guess I didn't take care of myself well enough.'"

The losses in the Early Transition, voluntary or involuntary—whether loss of persons or loss of place or loss of beloved possessions—form the tasks of that transition. Together they represent the loss of a way of life. But the issue is not whether or how many or which losses will be experienced; the issue is whether these losses will be so consuming as to obliterate purpose and reason for being. Does the Early Transition end in the ashes of loss or does the persona arise from the ashes once again? The answer is known only when the threshold is passed and the travelers have arrived at a new stage of life.

The Death of a Spouse or Partner

The most dramatic loss of the Early Transition involves the death of a spouse or partner.

> Sheila and Buddy hadn't really retired, they said; they just sold off the dairy herd so they had money and time to travel. That was about twenty years ago and now they were slowing down. More and more they talked about selling their acres and moving into town, but property values weren't so good and, anyway, this was home and their four grandkids still loved coming to the farm for a couple of weeks in the summer, "except that last year Yvonne and Kathy had backpacked in Thailand instead." Late in the winter Sheila felt so listless and just plain sick that she went to the clinic. The news was devastating. "Ovarian cancer," the doctor had said, "and it has spread to your lungs and lymph glands."

The last six months, Buddy now remembers, were unbelievably painful and intimate. After Sheila's death, Buddy spent many days with bouts of crying, thinking about his life with Sheila. When friends visited he always brought the conversation back to the question that haunted him: Why?

The loss of a partner or spouse is devastating in many ways. Day in and day out, often for many, many years, partners have shared their lives.

This is often intensified by the length of time we have spent with our partner. If we have been with our partner for many years, we may find that our partner completes our thoughts and is complementary in our actions. We are left feeling as if we have lost half of our self in addition to our partner. (Noel & Blair, 2002, Section 1)

The poignancy of this loss is often felt in the routines that are the fabric of daily life: one got up first and made the coffee, one made the bed; one cleaned the bathrooms, one cleaned the kitchen; one shopped for groceries, one usually cooked; one got in on this side of the bed, one on the other. The loss usually involves a significant other, a trusted companion, as well as a socially acceptable sexual partner. The significance of any of these roles varies, depending on the individual and the couple, and particularly on the roles and activities that they shared.

> When Jerry's doctor gave him six months to live, he and Estelle were devastated. It was literally the end of their world. After his death nearly eight months after the diagnosis, Estelle looked back on those months: "It was the happiest time. We got to know each other."

The death of a partner or spouse may impact the survivor in various ways. The one who remains may be financially jeopardized, may have to move, may be the one the children or others turn to for consolation, and will have to try to move forward alone, making new friends, new plans, a new life. This loss of a partner is unique and permanent (Noel & Blair, 2002, Section 1). According to Rappaport (2001), a drop in economic status accompanies widowhood, both because of individual decisions about retirement programs and resources and because of the allocation of survivor annuity and Social Security benefits (p. 4). Data obtained through the Older Couples Study revealed that 6 percent of widowed persons had serious financial problems following the death of a spouse, but 63 percent reported less income and 34 percent described a significantly increased financial strain (Utz, 2002). On the other hand, the dying spouse may have been overly demanding if not abusive, less than a loving or loved partner, and contributed to the dysfunctionality of the union. Or the dying partner may have lived too long, the victim of prolonged suffering, and a significant care burden.

The death of the spouse often happens over weeks and months, and grieving may begin when it becomes clear that the spouse is terminally ill or approaching the end of life. This process of grieving can be made all the more difficult by the pressure of care for the dying person, and the need to make the best possible care decisions. And in this time of intense grief, the ill partner may have little to offer by way of support. This is not always the case, but it is a frequent occurrence. One woman said, "It was devastating. Joyce just wasn't there for me when I needed her the most."

The tasks of the survivor, whether widow or widower, may seem overwhelming. At an emotional level, there is the giant challenge of coming to terms with the loss, accepting it, grieving it, finding meaning in it. At the physical level, there is the exhaustion that comes from physical and emotional exertion, no matter whether the death was unexpected, or whether it was the final result of months of suffering requiring extended caregiving. At the cognitive level, there are the myriad decisions to which attention must be given: settling an estate, seeing to one's own financial maintenance, responding to the initiatives of friends and relatives, and so on.

But in reality, these neat categories, outlining the emotional, physical, and cognitive, all merge with and obstruct one another. How can one attend to the affairs of the estate if one is busy grieving? And how can one grieve if one is caught up in fiscal matters? In addition, there is the need to maintain life's flow and rhythm: to maintain its relationships and continue its commitments, to receive support and continue life in community. Survivors may need assistance sorting out the tasks attendant upon surviving, and in particular they may need help in recognizing the importance of gaining strength in the face of exhaustion and gaining their equilibrium in the face of grief as critical survival tasks.

LOSS AND RECOVERY

Although the Early Transition leads to an ill-defined future, it is not without hope. There is the witness of others who have recovered from loss. Because they have endured loss and come back to a life of love and fulfillment, it is possible to trust that somehow the grief of the Early Transition will be neither permanent nor all-consuming. The pain may force a deep self-examination, there to discover new strengths. Or "it may also be that the pain keeps us open in our waiting—asking, listening, looking, willing to make that journey into self—a journey few of us undertake with any seriousness until compelled by our suffering" (O'Connor, 1987, pp. 14-15).

It may also force one, according to Attig (2001, pp. 33-34), back to those fundamental questions of identity and purpose. He describes this as "relearning the world," attaching meanings to old experiences and actions, reading new meanings into surroundings and events, and finding meaning in daily life patterns as well as long-held hopes and aspirations. New energy may be released as an outcome of successful mourning.

Paul Tournier (1983) in *Creative Suffering,* claims, "the greater the grief, the greater the creative energy to which it gives rise. . . . I can truly say that I have great grief and that I am a happy man" (p. 58).

After the death of his wife from cancer, C.S. Lewis (1961) described the gift of marriage as something "very close and intimate," but he noted that "there is spread over everything a vague sense of wrongness, of something amiss" (pp. 18, 30). But toward the end of that year there was for Lewis a moment of grace:

> Something quite unexpected happened. It came this morning early. For various reasons . . . my heart was lighter than it had been for many weeks. . . . Suddenly at the very moment when, so far, I mourned H. [his deceased wife] least, I remembered her best. Indeed it was something (almost) better than memory; an instantaneous unanswerable impression. To say it was like a meeting would be going too far. Yet there was something in it which tempts one to use those words. (p. 37)

To struggle against losses, as Yungblut (1990) says in *On Hallowing One's Diminishment,* is like Jacob wrestling with the angel—no one will get out of the struggle unmarked. But as Yungblut reflects, "It is well to see that, in doing so, one is struggling against an angel and not to let go until one has received the distinctive blessing of that particular angel" (p. 11). He points to the reality that in loss there is possible gain—a blessing, even. But few will see that before or during the trauma of the transition that ends Extended Middle Age.

Afterward there may appear some grace notes in the form of glimmers of light, moments of joy, times of relaxation. It may be that distance and perspective soften the sharp edges. There may be good recollections of people who helped, or the forgiveness expressed by a dying person, or a sense of freedom that the oppression of accumu-lated possessions has been lifted. The development of mature ego defenses and adaptive abilities may aid in embracing the new life cir-cumstances. Grace notes come in all forms: persons, memories, ex-pectations, and hopes. They may come in the release from the endless and consuming burden of caregiving, the uplift of friends new and old, or the promise held by one's future. Vaillant (2002) refers to this adaptation as the "capacity to turn lemons into lemonade and not to turn molehills into mountains" (p. 206).

Growth in Recovery

Evidence abounds of the resilience of persons as they undergo the changes of the Early Transition. Many examples suggest a prevailing mental and physical healthfulness during this time. A study directed by Laura Carstensen reported that "older people regulate their emotional states better than younger people" ("Elderly Show Their Emotional Know-How," 1999, p. 374). She noted that older adults experience richer mixes of feelings, but that positive emotions linger longer, and negative ones make briefer intrusions as adults age. Data from the Health and Retirement Study indicate that the percentage of persons with severe depressive symptoms decreases slightly between the age periods of 65 to 69 and 70 to 74, and then remains constant through age 79 for both men and women (*Older Americans 2000: Key Indica-tors of Well Being,* 2000).

An analysis of several studies related to feelings of physical well-being and health found that older persons feel good about life even when their physical conditions are not the best. These studies have concluded that subjective views of life satisfaction and well-being are more effective in explaining and predicting behavior and feelings than objective measures of health, income, or education (Rudinger & Thomae, 1990). What can be concluded from this research is that per-sonal perspective is more significant than the demographic variables that describe a person's circumstance. How one views one's situation is critical. Neither class nor health can predict happiness or despair. Recent research also suggests that persons' sense of self-efficacy contributes to their levels of life quality and satisfaction. In this study, widows benefited from self-efficacy in areas of interpersonal relations, emotional stability, and spiritual health, whereas widowers felt competent in areas of instrumental activity, financial security, and physical health. The author notes the positive role of spiritual health efficacy during difficult times (Fry, 2001). A critical component to the support of persons engaged in the Early Transition is helping them maintain their sense of empowerment and their role in decision making.

It is important to recognize that suffering, whether physical or emotional, carries different meanings for different people based on culture and religion. For many, it is a condition to be avoided and, if unavoidable, to be overcome. But for others, it is a religious phenomenon, a path to deeper faith and meaning, indeed to a participation in or with the divine, a condition to be treasured. Whatever the meaning associated with suffering, a life-threatening illness that happens to someone close to us "takes us into the underworld as a companion on a journey," taking us into our own depths of feeling and meaning "to the essence of who we are and what we are here for at a soul level. It is not just the patient but others who are tested by illness" (Bolen, 1996, p. 115). It is therefore appropriate for professionals and others who provide support during times of grief or trauma to probe a person's perception of the events and feelings being experienced in order to understand the significance being attached to them and the meaning derived from them.

Mary Pipher (1999) concludes that with physical decline comes psychological growth:

> With a failing body and a life filled with losses, a person can't help but think of the meaning of life. As there is more to accept, there is more capacity to accept. . . . As bodies become frail and vulnerable, souls often grow strong and resilient. (p. 216)

MEANING AND RELATIONSHIPS

Ken and Mary Gergen (2002) point to an important relationship between life meaning and relationships:

> What gives meaning to life in the later years? What provides the nourishment, zest and joy of daily living? In the middle years the answers were often obvious—romance, one's profession, raising children, moving up, dedication to a cause, and so on. But in the

later years many of the common answers cease to be relevant, and depression is a frequent result. . . . What is the key? At least one compelling possibility is that meaning/full endeavors spring primarily from relationships. It is through relationships that we negotiate good and evil, separate worth from worthless, and determine that certain activities are rewarding while others a waste of time. (p. 1)

Positively, this points to the value of relationships in a "meaning/full" life. As a challenge it points to the need to develop and maintain a broad range of relationships, including family members, close friends, and casual acquaintances. It also warns of the potential risks associated with the loss or death of a primary intimate relationship, a loss greatly exacerbated when that broad range of relationships is absent. The issue is powerfully linked to both age and gender.

The relationship need not be core to be sorely missed. Every network of colleagues and friends has its importance. Every new network of people who share commitments takes time and effort to build. Closeness takes time to develop. But the loss of a spouse or partner is uniquely devastating, and this is the paradox, the anomaly. Deep friendships are important. A stable marriage matters. The depth of engagement with a partner, the amount of self selflessly shared—the very things that make for a fine relationship will, in the moment of loss, deepen the pain. The death of a spouse can activate the most profound kind of grief, with many conflicting emotions—anger, powerlessness, relief, guilt, withdrawal, and isolation (Gergen & Gergen, 2002).

Social adjustments associated with late life bereavement may be one of the most difficult changes an older adult faces. In addition to the destruction of one's physical, emotional, and mental equilibrium, the loss of a spouse may also have a devastating impact on one's social network. The events preceding the death of a spouse may involve illness and incapacitation of varying duration, requiring extensive caregiving, and limiting involvement in social activities outside the home. The result is a drawing inward, a conservation of strength and resources, and a necessary constraint of interaction with one's social network. By the time of bereavement, interaction with one's social network may already be greatly curtailed. Following the loss of a spouse or partner, relationships with other married couples, formerly best friends, may become awkward with the realization that, as a single, one is something of a misfit. In addition to changing status from married to unmarried, survivors are challenged to reestablish and realign their social networks and to alter their social activities in ways that are appropriate and useful in their new status.

For some older men and women, making friends has been a natural and important component of their personalities. But for many married couples, one—usually the wife—has served as the "social secretary" whose role was to organize and maintain contacts with the social network. When the loss of a spouse is the loss of the social envoy, the remaining partner not only suffers the devastating loss of a spouse, but also the absence of a dependable bridge into the world of relationships. Conversely, with the loss of a husband, the wife, lacking a consistent male escort, may be consigned to the social network of singles and fellow widows. The survivor is left not only with a sense of loss, but also with the need to affirm the importance of relationships, and to create or recover the skills needed to establish and maintain the necessary social network and activities. Using data from the Changing Lives of Older Couples study, Rebecca Utz and others found that 87 percent of widowed people said they tried to keep busy or get involved in some activity as a way to cope with feelings of grief or loneliness, with the result that widowed men and women have higher levels of informal social participation than their nonwidowed peers, getting together with friends, neighbors, or relatives and talking on the phone more often than when their spouses were alive (Utz, Carr, Nesse, & Wortman, 2002).

Conversely, being alone is not the same as being lonely. Helen Hayes describes her change from the active life of a married actress to that of a retired widow: "Solitude—doing things alone—is one of the most blessed things in the world. The mind relaxes and thoughts begin to flow and I think I am beginning to find myself a little bit" (Kovol, 1973, as cited in Huyck & Hoyer, 1982, p. 395).

Persons with sufficient financial resources to sustain them in older adulthood often overlook the experience of those who lack resources. The picture is clouded by the fact that many of the resource poor are also members of an ethnic minority group, making it difficult to distinguish characteristics born of poverty from those born of ethnic tradition. For example, ethnic groups with their extended family and social networks provide a support system; these support systems consist of lineal, consanguineous, and fictive members, depending on the ethnic tradition. The construction of the network is likely to differ between African-American, Asian, and Hispanic groups. Similarly, poor families tend to be rich in kin networks as a response to the need for practical assistance. Furthermore, ethnic networks tend to serve as an integrative force and a compensatory buffer that assist in the adaptation of elderly members in older adulthood (Johnson, 1995, p. 307). Congregations and ethnically oriented community organizations also provide both a network of support as well as a setting for the exchange of goods and services among the poor. The forces of practicality and tradition tend to provide an in-place support system already in place when events leading to an Early Transition occur. But lest these statements constitute a kind of stereotype, more than one Native American elder has mourned the desertion of the "old ways" by children and grandchildren, more than one elderly black woman has been found in isolation, and another announced to one of the authors that "I want to go to a nursing home because I don't trust my kids to take care of me."

Life stories of gay Americans experiencing the Early Transition also illustrate alternative styles of relational support. In some locales, opportunities for socialization are restricted by antigay sentiments, and among some contact with families may be distant and support from them ranges from limited to nonexistent. At the same time, gays report that they receive emotional and physical support from a network of friends who assist with instrumental tasks, such as grocery shopping and transportation, not unlike the social support system provided by the heterosexual community (Brown, Alley, Sorosy, Quarto, & Look, 2000, p. 49).

DIFFERENCES AND SIMILARITIES

Of course, in all this, between one person's losses and another's, and one set of life circumstances and another, there are similarities and differences. Early Transition has some shared characteristics no matter who passes the threshold, but the differences in experience are so real as to merit attention.

A notable difference in the way people will experience Early Transition is whether or not the journey is entered into voluntarily, although there is, of course, always a certain degree of involuntariness in the Early Transition. Take this example:

> When Phil retired as chief accountant for a large metropolitan hospital, he and Marie sold their suburban home and built a new, large house in a small, midwestern resort community. They were active participants in the life and leadership of their new community for almost 15 years. Chronic but manageable health problems and the awareness that their children had located in the Pacific Northwest led them to a life-changing decision. They decided to sell their home and many of their possessions and locate in a retirement facility near their children and near good health care facilities. Their choices were deliberate, but not without tears and a certain sense of diminishment. The retirement apartment was comfortable, but barely half of the square footage of their former home. The volunteering they do now is only a shadow of the leadership roles they had played in their former community.

The voluntary dimension of this transition was that in their passage to their revised lifestyle Phil and Marie had made decisions for themselves and according to their own schedule. The involuntary dimension was their experience of chronic but manageable health problems and their children's decisions to relocate in the Pacific Northwest. Compare their experiences with these:

> At 79 Mo is a bit stooped, but still a giant of a man, as he comes into the YMCA gym and greets his 8 a.m. work-out pals. Six months ago his wife, Lucy, was diagnosed with a rare lung condition that affected her heart and kidneys. "It completely changed my life," Mo says without a shadow of self-pity. "I go home after the gym and stay home. I've given up going out to ball games, or anywhere without her. You know, you're just afraid what you might find when you went home if you stayed away too long." The little house they are in, with the big yard and now giant trees Mo himself planted when he got back from World War II, doesn't really fit their needs. "Maybe we'll move into a three-room place all on one floor. Stairs are bad for Lucy. She won't even go with me to bring up the gifts [at their church, during Mass]; she's afraid she wouldn't make it back to the pew."

Mo and Lucy are being pressed into a change mode by problems associated with Lucy's health. Although their time frame may be more compressed than that of Phil and Marie, decisions about housing, lifestyle, and purpose for both couples require choices from among many options as well as the time for a smooth transition. Not all transitions are so gentle or unrestrained.

> Susan is in the middle of a divorce. It came as a total shock to her; even now she is not sure she saw it coming. She has now known about "the other woman" for six months, since Ken made his announcement. She finds it hard to get to the practical issues, the hurt is so bad. Almost 44 years of marriage ending in this. But she tries to wrestle with legal and financial matters, and the older daughter's split allegiances—and access to her two precious grandchildren.

Differences in the experience of Early Transition result from a variety of interrelated factors: a person's age when the transition occurs, the social history a person carries by virtue of being born at a certain time, and other personal life circumstances.

The framework of this book downplays chronological age in favor of a model of transitions and stable periods. Yet, although age doesn't tell us everything, it tells us something. We expect different physical abilities in a person at age 27 than at age 72. And the person who comes to Early Transition at age 65 will have a different experience than the person who comes to it at age 78. In the examples just given, age—in the sense of where persons are on their life's journey—was a factor for Phil and Marie and for Mo and Lucy, as all were around 80 when the transition occurred. Mo put it this way: "I don't know if the good Lord meant us to live this long, but we carry on. What can you do?" People find themselves at a time in life when their energies go less into activities designed to "conquer the world" and more into maintaining a lifestyle that allows them to prevail and flourish in spite of losses. If they live long enough in Extended Middle Age, some may find themselves in Early Transition putting proportionally more energy into mourning and managing loss in order not to be overwhelmed and to live with choices and dignity.

Other differences derive from that time in history in which the life journey occurs. People bring with themselves attitudes and standards they learned growing up. For example, Susan's divorce may be related to her specific time in history. If she had been born a few decades earlier, it is less likely (although not unheard of) that she would have been divorced this late in life. People also bear the marks of historical events. For example, people who began life in 1920 had a different life course and, quite likely, different outcomes than people who began life in 1930 or in 1940.

And then there are personal life circumstances: personal choices, gender, socioeconomic status, ethnicity, birth order, and so on. In all the examples, personal life circumstances played a role. Socioeconomic status played a role in Phil and Marie's decisions; they had the personal and financial resources to move on. Compare their story with Edna's:

> I was exhausted. I was just so tired I couldn't keep going. George wandered and I had to keep an eye on him 24 hours a day; he forgot everything—we didn't have a real conversation in months; he was moody and sometimes I was afraid he was going to get violent. And he started wetting the bed four or five times a night. And every time he did, he wanted the bed changed. Everyone told me just use Depends. Sure. I'm 5'4" and I weigh 135 pounds and he's 6'2" and weighs 240. And I was going to put a diaper on him? People told me to put him in a nursing home. They cost $4,200 a month around here and all we have is this small house, George's pension, and Social Security. If George hadn't been hospitalized with a stroke and all those complications, I don't know where I would have turned. Thank God they didn't send him home. He's in the VA [Veterans Administration Hospital]. The doctors say he won't be coming home. But I don't think George much knows where he is now. And me, I'm just trying to put my life together and get on with it.

The complex interaction of contexts and relationships highlights differences in the way persons pass through threshold events. Personal life circumstances, many of which are beyond a person's control, are powerful elements in the different ways in which people go through Early Transition. The ability to plan appropriately may be limited by some of these circumstances.

But there are strong similarities in the ways in which persons go into that "betwixt and between" time of life that marks the end of Extended Middle Age. What they have in common is the end of a familiar life. The pattern of days and weeks and years gives way to a new and unsought after life pattern. There is a sense of transition, of passage, and a way through that is not clear. The demands of this journey through change are rigorous. It is, in a sense, a sort of boot camp to toughen up people to be older adults. Their gaze has turned from the middle years to life ahead. And however well they may be, death has their attention.

PREPARING FOR THE EARLY TRANSITION

What can one do to prepare for this transition? Or as a friend put it, "Is there useful homework?" A significant variable is whether or not the choice to embark on the Early Transition is self-initiated. An example of a self-initiated move is when a diminishment in personal resources, health, or well-being is recognized, and the decision to relocate, downsize, or change one's lifestyle is made on one's own schedule. In such cases, there can be preparation in the selection of a new place to live, in the engagement with new potential friends, in the process of paring down possessions to fit a new lifestyle, in plans for less strenuous but satisfying ways of mattering. But in another scenario, there may be little or no intentionality in the initiation or structure of the transition: we do not choose illness or death of a spouse, nor do we choose this dramatic change in our own capabilities. Instead, suddenly it is as Teilhard de Chardin (1960) wrote, "one of these processes of disorganization [that] has installed itself at the very heart of our lives" (p. 54).

In both cases the most basic preparation is long term—how to live, how to think about life and make choices, how to attend to what is around us, how to care for others, how to act responsibly even when growth is difficult, how to be in love. There are habits of body, mind, heart, and spirit that can make a difference in the way the drama of Early Transition is experienced.

Also, on a more mundane level, there are choices about where to live and how to pay for it that can help avoid "why didn't I do that a year ago" self-recriminations. The lives of others provide ample evidence that the failure to take initiative to choose the place to live that is most likely to give good support in aging has potentially high— and avoidable—costs. Optimally, persons can ask what kind of living situation will best support them in their aging. This process requires careful attention to the potential gains and losses of each choice, as well as careful attention to financial and human costs (MacBean & Simmons, 2006).

The role of the professional is to help those anticipating the Early Transition, as well as those engaged in it, to plan appropriately, to make decisions that advance individual purposes and values, to make the best use of their resources, to claim the freedom to become the persons they choose to be, to enjoy intimacy and weather loss, and, above all, to rebuild their enthusiasm for living. What becomes clear in the Early Transition is that each of these takes on new meaning and each will be, in its own way, a new challenge as individuals regain sensitivity to the gifts recognized and the wonders of the worlds shared, even in the face of loss.

Chapter 5

An Older Adult Lifestyle

The changes of the Early Transition often impose dramatic changes for older adults in the way life is viewed and lived. But having experienced, indeed suffered, such major alterations can life proceed? Can transformation come out of transition? Can hope for the rest of life come forth from trauma? Can dreams still be fulfilled? The answer that this chapter gives to these and all such questions is yes—an affirmation of the experience of many who have gone through this transition and a recognition of the amazing resilience of so many older adults.

Professionals who serve older adults often find that the need that they are called upon to address at this particular juncture is to assist their clients in coming to that yes. In supporting the work of professionals and family members, this chapter takes as its premise that older adults who have passed the Early Transition, whatever their losses, still have great potential for growth, happiness, and active well-being.

WHO SURVIVED?

Those described here are those who have passed a milestone from which there is no return. They are those who have grieved the loss of a spouse; those who have suffered the loss of their own health and well-being or that of their partner; those who have given up the comfort of familiar surroundings for a new place; those who have voluntarily traded in a middle-age lifestyle for one befitting a person in the later years; or those who have reduced, curtailed, or otherwise diminished

A Journey Called Aging: Challenges and Opportunities in Older Adulthood
© 2007 by The Haworth Press, Taylor & Francis Group. All rights reserved.
doi:10.1300/5915_06   *115*

aspects of their activity or lifestyle. Middle age has been irretrievably left behind. The impact has been psychological as well as physical, jarring self-concept, self-worth, and social well-being, and challenging any naively sanguine view of the future. Some are convinced that they have exhausted their resources and completely depleted their resilience.

Only an unfeeling person would minimize the impact of any of these events. For some, the grief may appear too overwhelming, the suffering too consuming, or the relocation too disorienting to imagine any future, let alone one that offers fulfillment. Nevertheless this period following the Early Transition represents a time in which one's life is re-created through the continued process of meaning-making, the exercise of choices, the pursuit of relationships, and the courage to anticipate and stand in the face of future transitions. This will be the time of "settling in" to older adulthood, a time when older adults see themselves as an integral part of the older population and socialize with others like themselves.

The chronological age at which some precipitating event occurs will color the identification with the older adult population. For example, a woman who becomes a widow at the age of 70 is likely to struggle with different issues in identifying with the older adult population than her older sister who is widowed at age 80. The differences are real. The self and social perceptions that one's lot is now cast with the older adult population are also real. Ethnic and cultural traditions, socioeconomic status, and gender are all important determinants of how a person "settles in" to older adulthood; they are not, however, determinants of either the satisfaction or fulfillment that accompany successful aging.

For some people, the process will be adaptive: that is, they will come to terms with their new situation and will make the necessary modifications and accommodations to adjust to it. For others, the process will be transformative and will involve a conversion of both the person and the situation into something new.

The Demographic Data

Another way to describe those in this period is to review pertinent demographic data. The nondisabled older adult population has increased steadily from 1982 through 1999: three major findings of the

National Long Term Care Survey are "(i) an acceleration of the decline in chronic disability prevalence from 1994 to 1999 compared with 1989 to 1994, (ii) the large relative and absolute drop in institutional use, and (iii) disability decline for black Americans after 1989" (Manton & Gu, 2001, p. 6357). Although the decline is distributed across the older adult population, it has increased with age, with more dramatic declines in both the 75 to 84 and 85 plus age groups, indicating that this decline in disability is very likely to have occurred among those in the Older Adult Lifestyle period.

One implication of this decline is that proportionately fewer older adults in this period will live in nursing-home facilities, with those experiencing disability opting instead to remain in their homes or receive care in residential-care apartment complexes or assisted-care living facilities. The percentage of the population from 75 to 84 years living in nursing homes declined from 6.1 percent in 1990 to 4.7 percent in 2000 (Hetzel & Smith, 2001, p. 8).

Life expectancy for the overall population reached new highs at the beginning of this century, with an average life expectancy at birth of 77.2 years, and increased for both men and women as well as whites and blacks. For men, life expectancy increased to 74.4 years and women to 79.8 years. (However, preliminary indicators suggest that this gap may be narrowing.) Given this continuing decline in the death rate, persons in their midseventies may expect to live an average of 11 plus additional years—10.2 years for white men and 12.3 years for white women, 9.3 years for black men and 11.7 years for black women (Centers for Disease Control and Prevention, 2001b, Table 7). Declining disability and decreased mortality rates suggest that more persons than previously are likely to live into their eighties and beyond, while maintaining autonomy, self-care, and an active lifestyle. Many of these will be people who have transitioned through loss to an Older Adult Lifestyle.

Correlations are evident between disability and mortality rates and certain demographic variables. For example, disability declined by a greater percentage for blacks than for nonblacks over the 1989 to 1999 period (Manton & Gu, 2001). On the other hand, death rates and life expectancy tables show that whites in their midseventies are likely to live approximately one year on average longer than blacks. However, the death rate for the Hispanic population during the years

70 to 74 is lower than for either the white or black populations (Arias, Anderson, Kung, Murphy, & Kochanek, 2003, Table 4).

Shaping the Older Adult Experience

Within broad, nationwide generalizations, data describing life expectancy, health, and disability are shaped by race, gender, age, class, education, and place. Race and place intersect with age in particular ways in the inner city, as Katherine Newman (2003) points out in *A Different Shade of Gray: Midlife and Beyond in the Inner City*. Another study (Murray, Michaud, McKenna, & Marks, 1998) found that life expectancy in the United States varies dramatically by county. For example, residents of counties with significant American Indian populations have very low average life expectancies. This is also true of counties in Arkansas, Mississippi, and Louisiana in the Mississippi Delta, as well as several urban inner-city areas. The counties with the highest life expectancies are mostly rural midwestern or western counties in Minnesota, South Dakota, Iowa, Colorado, Montana, and Utah. The authors point to a high correlation between these findings and levels of income and education, but they admit that anomalies exist where high life expectancy occurs in areas of low income and low rates of educational attainment.

Individual experience during the youth and adult years also shapes the Older Adult Lifestyle period. Unemployment and underemployment during the adult years, the sacrifice of income or marriage for caregiving, and the exhaustion of resources for family emergencies leave a legacy of hardship in the years after the losses of the Early Transition. Low income and meager savings in adulthood often translate into poverty in older adulthood. According to Rank and Hirschl (1999),

> 40 percent of America's elderly population will experience a year below the poverty line at some point between the ages of 60 and 90, and 48 percent of elders will experience poverty at the 125 percent level. . . . The likelihood of elderly Americans ever encountering a year below the poverty line increases dramatically for those who are Black, not married, and/or who have less than 12 years of education. (p. S184)

Persons arriving at this period are more likely to be women who on average will live their final 15 years as widows (Carstensen, 2001, p. 267). A similar population are women who sought employment after divorce in their forties and fifties and, having not worked long enough to build a secure pension, have either to continue working or subsist with limited resources (Uchitelle, 2001). According to the U.S. Census Bureau (2003a, Table 2), 55 percent of the female population 75 to 84 years of age are widows, compared with 18.4 percent of the male population the same age; 6.7 percent are divorced or separated, compared to 5.6 percent of males; and 3.2 percent were never married, compared with 4.0 percent of males. This statistic—that 65 percent of women and 28 percent of men between the ages of 75 and 84 are unmarried—foregrounds all others and provides this period with its most prominent feature.

The experience of each older person will combine the sweeping generalities of demographic variables (age, gender, race, and ethnicity) with the more specific aspects of individual experience (education, income, marital status, and genetic heritage) to shape the experience in older adulthood of each person. Anticipation of any future will take both into account.

But common to all who have made the transition described in the preceding chapter is the need to pick up the pieces of one's life following the transition. This involves reorganizing the tasks of daily living, and planning and implementing the next steps to be taken. Then there is the future: What will it look like now that the present is different? Of course, there is always the temptation to pretend that, despite the transition, nothing has changed. The circumstances say otherwise. To quote Carl Jung (1933):

> [W]e cannot live the afternoon of life according to the programme of life's morning—for what was great in the morning will be little at evening, and what in the morning was true will at evening have become a lie. (p. 108)

A new program—a new compass, even a new or renewed self? This agenda of redefinition serves as the context for both the professional and the family relationship with a person in the Older Adult Lifestyle period. The dominant themes that frame the interaction of persons in this period with the professionals who serve them and the family and friends who love them are themes of rediscovering and re-creating identity, intimacy, and generativity, to use Erikson's (1950) language, or addressing the basic questions of "Who am I? What will I do? With whom will I do it?"

REINVENTING THE SELF

Stanley Kunitz (2000) captures this sense of looking back while moving forward, the continuity between survival and rebirth:

I have walked through many lives,
some of them my own,
and I am not who I was,
though some principle of being
abides, from which I struggle
not to stray.* (p. 217)

As Kunitz makes eloquently clear, these people are not who they were when they entered older adulthood. But who are they? Many metaphors describe this process in which new life comes from the old, plants grow out of the cold earth, spirits are reborn, fire arises from ashes, and so on. This chapter has already described the process in terms of adaptation or transformation. Mark Gerzon (1992) depicts the experience as a metamorphosis, recalling the caterpillar spinning its cocoon and coming forth as a butterfly (p. xiv). The phrase "rein-venting the self" emphasizes two notions: first, that the re-created self, born out of the old, has both continuity and newness, and, sec-ond, that the responsibility for the process rests with the individual. Hence the challenge: How does one go about being a helper or a friend through the reinventing process?

Unfamiliar and awkward as the word "reinvent" may sound, neither the idea nor the experience is really new. Most individuals, young and old, have reinvented themselves through a number of identities. They have been siblings, newlyweds, students, parents, grandparents, factory workers, ministers, teachers, salespeople, program directors, service industry employees, professionals of all sorts, and volunteers, all in one lifetime. The story of these lives is one of reinventing the self, re-creating identities, personages, and purposes to meet new challenges, building on the experience and other resources available, and devoting these to address needs then current. Reinventing balances the old with the new, anchoring new ventures in a continuity with the past, creating something new that is nonetheless recognizable as a continuation of the old.

A person with many diverse life experiences recalls this evolution in his life (Terkel, 1995):

> What I'm doing now is a continuation of my life. I've had about four lives. Retirement is my fifth. Childhood in Oregon, Commonwealth College. Working with the children of miners in West Virginia. I took a ball, bat, and bicycle into the coal camps and organized clubs for the kids. I was down in North Carolina, during the bitter textile strike, working with the children. In St. Louis, I was helping organize the unemployed. I became educational director of the UEWA (United Electrical Workers of America), Midwestern district. Four years in the army. Then came Chicago and carpentry. Now is my fifth—or is it sixth?—life. (p. 251)

Sharon Kaufman (1986) describes how

> people formulate and reformulate personal and cultural symbols of their past to create a meaningful, coherent sense of self, and in the process they create a viable present. In this way, the ageless self emerges: its definition is ongoing, continuous, and creative. (p. 14)

If one is a widow, having been a wife who derived her identity or her income in whole or part from her husband, she is now called upon to reformulate her identity as a single person. If one had been a robust, healthy, assertive individual who is now incapacitated by disease, then one must build a viable identity given these new and challenging circumstances. If for whatever reason the Early Transition required an individual or a couple to relocate into a new community or a new neighborhood, the focus must be on creating an identity in a new environment.

In some situations, particularly in certain ethnic groups, some roles—for example, that of widow—are traditionally defined with a range of expectations regarding dress, socialization, timeline, place of residence, and so on. In most instances, however, this transformation has no clear guidelines: the colors of the butterfly to come forth from the cocoon are chosen by the one who comes forth.

Setting Directions

The best way to set direction may be to ask key questions. In many situations, this becomes an important role of a professional, whether a physician, an attorney, a counselor, a social worker, or a pastor. Or an older adult may think of it as participating in an interview with the self about the future. Perhaps this dialogue with the self or with another sounds like an academic exercise or a fill-in-the-blanks test to an older person. But key questions must be asked: What has given your life the most meaning? What are the common threads woven throughout all that has happened to you? What in your life is important for you to affirm? What are you content to forget? What needs press most upon you in the present? Are these needs personal or are they the needs of the community or society? Are there significant persons, friends, or family whom you must consider or whom you wish to incorporate into your plans for your future? Can you draw a picture of yourself in two years or in five years? Can you distinguish your dreams from your expectations? Which will you follow?

Where lifelong desires and latent plans exist, they may be brought to the fore by loss and change and become the agenda for the reinvented lifestyle. This process begins in the dialogue with the self around the question "Who do I choose to be in the present circumstance?" The self, after a time of uncertainty, gets in touch with unfulfilled hopes and unachieved goals and puts these in the context of present-day needs, challenges, and opportunities.

For some, the examination of the self may be troublesome, probing hidden areas, requiring extended consideration, forcing difficult choices. Some answers do not come quickly, or easily. Failing to answer any of these in a moment is not tantamount to failing older adulthood. The questions probe some of the deep recesses of a person's values, testing the anchors to which lives are chained, and at the same time inquiring into circumstances and challenges that confront one on a daily basis. Parts of the inquiry may be painful, even threatening. It is this juxtaposition of experience of the past with experience of the present and how it is understood that sets the agenda for a revised lifestyle, fashioned around a reinvented person. The outcome is meaning and purpose, a life worth living and caring about.

In redirecting a life out of care and purpose, a retired health care administrator, following the loss of her husband after a long and difficult illness, saw an urgent need for better information and personal support for those facing health-related problems. This led her to volunteer as a parish nurse in an downtown parish. An attorney, after the loss of her mother for whom she was caregiver, speaks of her anger at how older men and women are treated in the workforce, as organizations force them into retirement. This led her into paths of advocacy. A businessman, after the forced sale of his own firm, assists new business ventures with their business plans. A retired factory worker lives with his daughter and son-in-law and sees his grandchildren off to school in the morning and greets them when they come home in the afternoon. He can't think of anything he would rather do. A person who has had many jobs fulfills his lifelong dream by opening a ceramics studio at the age of 80.

Of course, not all plans are as ambitious as these. Limitations imposed by health, resources, location, and other factors reduce some dreams to what is possible. Traveling to exotic places on the other side of the globe may give way to day trips and train travel because long flights make legs swell and bodies cramp. Simple activities, such as gardening, canning and preserving food for later consumption, going to local ballroom and square dances, all provide activity without costly expense for some, as does "getting together with the guys" or "getting together with the gals." Involvement in a nearby senior center may provide a wide range of opportunities for purposeful activity and supportive interaction with other persons of the same age at a modest cost. Earlier decisions about living in an attractive location, such as the Sunbelt, may be revised in favor of living close to family. Useful advice may be simplify, prioritize, and do.

Sometimes the challenges of the present combined with the uncertainty of the future lead one to live in the past. For some, memories are painful; for others, they provide a haven of refuge. Bertam Cohler (1993) distinguishes between "having an ever-enlarging past that conditions our present and to which we apprentice ourselves" and becoming master of the past (p. 200). Laurence McCullough (1993) describes the past as having the "power to arrest some lives, to bring them to a stop, without death occurring." He calls this "arrested aging" (p. 185). Re-creation looks forward from the past, claiming purpose and setting direction amid both challenge and uncertainty.

Thus a person is renewed by a process of self-examination, goal setting, engagement in community life, and interaction with others. Life will not reinvent anyone. The older person will grow and change and mature as plans are worked and continually adjusted to overcome the obstacles and take advantage of the opportunities encountered along the way.

In reinventing the self, the need and the strategy is to discover what the person wants most to do and what the world or the community needs most to have done. It is where a person's joy and the world's pain meet that provides the greatest opportunity to make a difference (Buechner, 1973, p. 95). Gail Sheehy (1995) advises that "it's not just having something to live for, but finding something you *have* to live for" (p. 421, emphasis added). Compelling needs range from family obligations (seeing a nephew through college) to personal accomplishments to making a contribution to the well-being of the community, or the world.

A recent theory of aging associates longevity not only with nurturing behavior during fertility (the classic theory) but also involving "intergenerational transfers to be made to others" (Lee, 2003, p. F3). New evidence suggests that responding to compelling needs also helps one to live longer.

Out of answers to the question "What do I choose to be in the present circumstances?" emerges a purpose for the future. The question may be wrestled within the quiet of the soul, it may be broached with a helping professional, or it may evolve in dialogue with the environment in which one lives and a conversation with the community of which one is a part, or in which one is seeking.

Reinventing Oneself

One strategy for discovery of a new self is reinventing oneself as a student. Groups of every stripe provide people for talking and listening, and activities to engage the mind and body. Following the death of her husband, Francine enrolled in classes to learn basic reading and writing skills. Her husband had always done the reading and writing for both of them. Now the responsibility fell to her alone. And besides, she had promised herself that someday she would study for her high school diploma. Now was that day as she reinvented herself as a student. Larry made a similar promise when circumstances required him to drop out of college during the Great Depression. After a successful career directing the operations of a large manufacturing firm, and after the death of his wife, he came to the campus of a large urban university with one goal in mind: "to get my degree." Graduation came, and with it an honor cord, as well as the notoriety that comes when an 84-year-old achieves his lifelong educational goal: a bachelor of science degree. Others have reinvented themselves as students through Elderhostel, Institutes for Learning in Retirement, programs in colleges and universities where older adults can audit courses at little or no cost, and educational travel designed especially for older persons. And many have engaged in self-directed learning, following their own interests and choosing their own methods. All have engaged in the process of learning by coping with the emotional, physical, cognitive, and spiritual changes that have occurred and will continue.

An important ancillary consequence of reinventing oneself as a student is that learning—"exercising the brain"—may provide several instrumental benefits: Several studies suggest that it serves as a deterrent to neurodegenerative disease (Nussbaum, 2001). Others (Fisher, 1986, 1998) link continued participation in learning activities with strategies that maintain effective memory usage as well as important occasions for socialization. And still others assume the role of student as a preparatory step toward other pursuits—a new career or hobby in retirement or simply the fulfillment of a desire to be expert or at least well informed about some topic or other.

Another important strategy for reinventing the self is through volunteering. Motives for volunteering range from socializing, to using one's time constructively, to making a difference. Most volunteers would agree that they benefit from the experience as much as do those whom they serve. For many volunteers in the Older Adult Lifestyle period, this role substitutes both for the work that consumed adulthood and for the play that may have been the focus of Extended Middle Age. Reinventing oneself as a volunteer may be a misnomer in many cases. These are lifelong volunteers who have simply grown older and who are now in the Older Adult Lifestyle period. Even for them, where volunteering becomes a new and major focus of life and the self, it can help in reinventing the self. It may involve the person in a nurturing role, compensating for reduced family responsibility, or as a leisure substitute. Volunteer activities provide structure as well as purpose: ancillary benefits of volunteering, in addition to "making a difference" and "being with other people," include regular obligations that provide a routine around which other activities may be scheduled as well as an important link to the community.

Volunteering available through a range of nonprofit organizations provides opportunities that appeal to the diverse interests of a heterogeneous population, from taking care of the environment to caring for children, from providing direct service at a food pantry to drafting a business plan for a new service agency.

Others reinvent themselves as family caregivers or, more accurately, are reinvented as they are thrust into this role as the result of the illness or disability of a spouse or other family member. One-fourth of all informal caregivers are between the ages of 65 and 75 years, and another 10 percent are at least 75 years of age. Approximately 72 percent of all informal caregivers are female, and an estimated 85 percent of caregivers are related to the recipient (Profile of Informal and Family Caregivers, n.d.). Conversely, according to Johnson and Wiener (2006),

> the community-based disabled population is sizeable. In 2002, about 8.7 million people age 65 and older living at home, or 26.5 percent of the population, reported some type of disability that limited their ability to perform basic personal activities or live independently. About 6.1 percent, or 2.0 million people, were severely disabled. (p. vii)

Larry Polivka (2005) claims that there is "an inescapably religious dimension to the caregiving experience. The self-sacrifice entailed in caregiving may be the closest brush with transcendence that most people will ever experience" (p. 561).

An increasing number of grandparents find themselves with responsibility as primary caregivers or surrogate parents to their own grandchildren. In 2000, 7.1 percent of those grandparents with responsibility for their grandchildren were age 70 to 79, and 1 percent were age 80 and above (U.S. Census Bureau, 2003b, p. 8). In some instances, major caregiving roles are short term, but for others, it becomes a new way of life.

Some reinvent themselves as paid workers, usually part-time, but with a rationale similar to that of the volunteer, except with the added benefit of a paycheck. The retired statistician who clerks at the gift shop, the retired industrial arts teacher who stocks shelves at the hardware store, the retired repairman who tests the water for a local utility, the retired factory worker who works as a part-time custodian at a church—each builds a new persona on a lifetime of skills. Others reinvent themselves as paid workers out of necessity. For some, financial resources have diminished in their adequacy; for others, the cost of health care has necessitated securing employment with health insurance benefits or a new income stream to help offset rising health care costs.

Reinventing at this time of life has parameters and requirements that differ from person to person, and that differ from earlier recreations of the self. For some, earning an income is no longer important; for others, the need to supplement the Social Security check is paramount. Many are driven by the need to repay someone or something for their own good fortune. For some, the use of well-honed skills or involvement with old friends in traditional activities in a familiar location meets their need. For others, the novel, the adventurous, the unfamiliar, even the bold and daring, claim their attention. Recounting his boyhood, former President Carter (2001) describes how his mother in her seventies, a new widow, joined the Peace Corps, not something expected of an older lady from Georgia, with the request that she be sent "where people have dark skins and need a nurse's service" (p. 267). A friend, unable to deal with the sorrow associated with her husband's death, returned to school to learn to be a grief counselor. In meeting her own immediate needs, she launched herself on a new career. Carolyn Heilbrun (1997) reminds of the danger of being "trapped in one's body and one's habits, not to recognize those supposedly sedate years as the time to discover new choices and to act upon them" (p. 35). Above all else, the reinvented self must meet needs for meaning and give a purpose for living that fits both the inventor and the time. It must also provide for socialization and satisfaction as well as meet expectations for fulfillment.

When asked why it is good to be old, May Sarton responded that she is more herself now than she has ever been. She is happier, more balanced, and more able to use her power, and there is less conflict. She concludes her statement: "I am surer of what my life is about, have less self-doubt to conquer" (Heilbrun, 1997, pp. 6-7). Reinvention of the self helps one be specific about what one may look forward to.

Maintaining the Self

Just as important as reinventing is maintaining one's health of body, mind, and spirit. This is a new challenge, particularly if the years of Extended Middle Age had ways of attending to health that are no longer appropriate or accessible. For the widow or widower, early morning walks with a spouse must be replaced by other kinds of activities or partnerships. For the now physically handicapped or challenged, vigorous cycling or hiking must give way to new ways of maintaining physical fitness at a level as high as possible.

Maintaining oneself is much more prosaic than re-creating oneself, but just as important, in the same way that periodic oil changes are not as exciting as checking out the new car models, but necessary if an auto is to function smoothly. Self-maintenance involves the upkeep of the components of the self—both the body and the mind—through periodic checkups, regular and frequent exercise, and occasional upgrades. Most people don't need to be reminded of the importance of regular physical checkups to keep those diseases that often afflict older adults at bay. The enemy is less the aging process than the diseases that both shorten life and diminish well-being.

With remarkable frequency, research findings underline the diverse positive outcomes of aerobic exercise, from lowering blood pressure and the risk of coronary artery disease to the strong possibility of generating new brain cells, increasing overall cognitive ability, improving short-term memory, and lowering the risk of getting Alzheimer's disease. All that, plus looking and feeling better at the same time.

For many, the challenge is to incorporate physical exercise into a schedule filled with other pursuits. Sometimes motivation increases when exercise occurs with others, either an individual on a walk, or a group for a workout or swim. The boredom that some experience may be ameliorated by combining socialization with exercise as well as by varying the exercise activities. There are new things to be tried: the septuagenarian who started lifting weights for the first time; the octogenarian who entered his first marathon; the administrative assistant who retired from her desk chair to her couch, but then took up bicycle riding with her grandchildren, only to become addicted to her bike as *the* way to get around.

Studs Terkel recounts the story of an older man who every morning at sunup would jump up and begin his farm work. When asked why he shouldn't be getting his rest, he replied, "Oh, if I didn't do that, this old body of mine would think I was through with it, and that would be the end of me" (Terkel, 1995, p. 400).

But good maintenance doesn't end with keeping the muscles and joints in shape. It also includes the mind and spirit. Accounts of decline in cognitive ability among older adults are vastly overestimated. Not only does it come later chronologically than previously believed, but most of the measured decline comes in two areas: the slowing of reaction time and the weakening of the ability to solve problems that are unrelated to an individual's experience. The good news about mental function, whether reasoning or remembering, is that intellectually stimulating activities help to keep the mind sharp (Schaie, 1994).

For someone in the Older Adult Lifestyle period, there may be very specific skills to master, particularly if household tasks had been divided along gender lines. New skills may also be required if the Early Transition involved relocation to a new setting. These activities may consist of managing one's own affairs, balancing the checkbook, managing investments, keeping a detailed schedule book, overseeing home maintenance requirements, learning to use public transportation, engaging in an active correspondence, whether with pen and paper or by computer. Men widowed in the Early Transition may need to learn culinary and homemaking skills, or develop the art of constructing a social calendar. Where there is some disability or specific chronic illness, even more skills may need to be honed in finding others who are faced with similar challenges, searching out the best research, making informed decisions about treatment, negotiating the insurance and Medicare mazes, lobbying for funding for research and advocacy, and supporting others whose health outcomes may be even more fragile.

The need to maintain the spirit is equally critical. For some, maintenance of the spirit is a religious activity and involves participation in the life of a religious institution or community. For others, it is the product of stimulating relationships, meaningful activities, possibly reading and meditation, and personal discipline.

The consequences of neglecting one's spiritual and emotional health, however, are just as severe as neglecting the physical or the cognitive. Depression may be born out of grief, loneliness, or despair; it may be exacerbated by or occur as the result of physical illness; and it may severely limit an individual's ability to function. The American Psychological Association (2003) estimates that as many as 20 percent of older adults in the community may suffer from depression. Depression among older adults has also become a significant predictor of suicides among this population (National Institute of Mental Health, 2003). Maintenance of mental health, particularly as it relates to depression, may involve treatment by a physician. The need to maintain a high level of physical and mental health is an important part of the agenda at this new place in life, using approaches that assist one to function optimally in solving the problems of living.

THE OTHERS IN LIFE

The activity of reinventing the self is every bit a social activity. Reinvention as a two-way street involves important others both as companions on the journey and co-conspirators in the creation and presentation of the new self. At the same time, reinvented relationships become the product of a reinvented self. Friends keep persons informed about their identity. They mirror the self in the process of creating and re-creating. As Martin Buber (1937) affirmed in his book *I and Thou,* a person's humanity is not an individual possession but is the product of a relationship, arising from the space between the self and another. At a more pragmatic level, one thinks of support, help in case of need, someone to call, no matter what, no matter when.

For some, this will be the first time in their lives when they have lived alone. As an older adult confessed, "There is this time when you wish you had somebody to lean on, you wish you had somebody to talk to, and you know that other people are just going to think you're whining."

Making New Friends

Someone has said that the secret to good marketing is "location, location, location." That is, being at the right place is critical to selling goods or providing a service. It is also critical to renewing friendships and creating new relationships. It also helps placing oneself in situations where one is likely to meet persons with similar interests, possibly the same age, who are also open to being friends. The secret to exploring potential friendships is remembering that while a person may be there to meet others, others are there for a similar purpose. Wendy Lustbader (2001) shares the story of a proud businessman, down on his luck, who landed in a subsidized apartment, much against his wishes. But after ten years, he claimed that his neighbors were the best friends he ever had. She comments that "once he discovered the power of kindness, first by receiving it and then by giving it many times over, he missed no opportunities." Shortly before his death, he said, "Nothing I attained as a successful businessman comes close to what I've gained here, in my supposed poverty" (pp. 202-203).

Just how critical it is to make new friends is caught in the remark of a recently widowed friend: "The worst thing about being my age is that my friends have all died." Her affirmation is supported by research (Carstensen, 2001, p. 266) that found that most friends in the latter years are friends of many years. What she didn't say was that the task of making new friends required commitment, energy, and thought.

This may be especially true where the specific pathway through the Early Transition was a physically debilitating illness or handicap for oneself or one's spouse. For example, some volunteer activities will not lend themselves well to certain physically handicapping conditions. And, for the partner supporting one with Alzheimer's, for example, particularly in a resource-poor community, the challenges for making friends may be daunting.

Making new friends may also be a challenge when one has relocated into more affordable housing in an urban area, as in the following account:

> Her children moved Minnie from the suburban family home into a small downtown apartment so that she would not have to "worry about the house." Since she could no longer drive, she would also be closer to the cultural events she loved to attend. At first, Minnie had to learn where to shop, how to use the buses, and what services were available to persons in her area. But making friends was the hardest. At first, she attended a nearby church, and later volunteered to help the priest minister to shut-ins in the neighborhood. She began washing her clothes more often than before in order to talk with other residents in the laundry room. Later, she posted an invitation on the bulletin board for others to join her in a shopping expedition to a mall on the other side of the city. More recently, she has volunteered to assist at the food pantry two blocks away in order to meet others from her neighborhood.

Minnie's story has not ended. Even as she nears the end of the Older Adult Lifestyle period, she continues to be vigilant in her desire to make friends and cultivate relationships.

No matter what the espoused objective of a program catering to an older adult audience, whether religious, educational, social service, or recreational, the underlying objective of most of its members is socialization. In one study, more participants in educational activities said they attended for reasons of socialization than to meet educational goals (Fisher, 1986). Groups also provide support for the lifestyle and goals of the reinvented self. The Kreitlows (1989) have found that one of the most important factors in a positive retirement is associating with others.

As part of their revised lifestyles, John got a part-time job in a hardware store, and Irv is employed three days a week as a bagger in the local grocery. Neither needs the money, but both need the opportunities for meeting people and interacting with colleagues that the part-time employment affords. Irv lists the friends who regularly shop on the days when he works and always check out through his lane. On his way home from swimming and exercising at the YMCA, Mac stops at a small local restaurant to buy a paper and coffee. He will consume both on the premises, along with conversation with other older men and women who appear most mornings for breakfast and conversation. *The New York Times* reported how six older women from Queens gather five times each week to play cards and have done so for 20 years (Fein, 1994, p. A16). Susan, on the other hand, wouldn't miss her church's breakfast study group every Thursday morning. The study is useful, challenging some of her pet ideas and supporting others, but what is really important is that she meets many her age, most of them widowed like herself. It is a comfortable group—so much so that she is considering asking some of the women she meets there to be travel companions on her next trip.

The experience of relocation, common to many in this period, may provide a convenient occasion for engaging new acquaintances, especially if the move is to a community that provides organized program activities. As part of a new environment, one may discover planned discussions of books or current events, games, interesting speakers who stimulate serious thought, or fellow residents who share thought-provoking ideas. But proximity does not guarantee a relationship that is productive of trust, affection, and support. No matter what the setting, the adage "To make a friend, be a friend" still applies.

Researchers have found that loneliness is a particular problem among members of the older gay and lesbian community where members tend to rely on long-standing friendship networks that have, over time, been disrupted by illness and death (Berger & Kelly, 2000, pp. 60-81). Expanding social networks often depends on the permeability of the boundaries of a social community.

Particular obstacles may be present with that 1.6 percent of persons over 65 who speak no or limited English at all and whose social contacts are thereby limited to persons speaking their language (U.S. Census Bureau, 2000a, Summary File 3—Sample Data, p. 19). In some instances, they reside in enclaves of individuals and families who share a common language and culture; in others, they reside in relative isolation and have limited opportunities for interaction, making the development of relationships through ordinary channels virtually impossible.

Enhancing Relationships

Finding new friends and establishing new relationships is only half the task. The other half consists in infusing new life and creativity into the relationships that currently exist—friends as well as family members. One place to begin is in considering the benefits of already established friendships.

The task of enhancing relationships requires a frank appraisal of the benefits a relationship provides, and, of equal importance, those benefits friends anticipate and enjoy from the relationship. Given such an assessment, the task of enhancement is to discover ways in which both parties benefit.

Fortunately, there are countless illustrations of persons possessing strength of character or other resources who reach out to individuals needing help or support—with no expectation of any return. Many work in programs, delivering meals or providing transportation as volunteers. But many more are simply good neighbors and good friends—giving back, providing services, sharing love, responding to obvious needs. Whatever the motivation, one cannot disregard the treasured relationships that grow out of the many times when love is shared and no return is expected.

Nor should one discount the ancillary benefits that may come from such activity. Recent research using data from the Changing Lives of Older Couples sample indicates that mortality was significantly reduced among older adults who reported providing instrumental support to friends, relatives, and neighbors, and older adults who reported providing emotional support to their spouses (Brown, Nesse, Vinokur, & Smith, 2003). Those who reported receiving support enjoyed no such effect; only those who gave it enjoyed reduced mortality. Instrumental support was defined as helping with transportation, errands, shopping, housework, child care, or other tasks. Emotional support was defined as helping another feel loved and cared for and being willing to listen.

Family Relationships

Family relationships present a somewhat different challenge. In some families, the unfolding of relationships—siblings, spouses, children, in-laws, grandchildren, and other relatives—has occurred in a healthy fashion, consistently open to include and respect other members. But in other families, relationships present a complicated tangle that has a way of continuing without resolution. It is hard to imagine a more important task of this period than addressing elements of this tangle so that whatever unfinished family business that exists may be completed.

Although not all knots of the tangle can be unraveled and not every relationship can be made perfect, that should not be an excuse for postponing activity designed to bring about reconciliation and harmony among these relationships. The passing of time, its healing properties, enhanced maturity of individuals, the awareness of mortality—all increase the potential for resolving difficulties and enhancing concord, so that here also the benefits of a relationship may increase to become significantly greater than the costs as the result of reconciliation. Where people have suffered severe violations of love and trust in the intergenerational families, the help of a professional who specializes in multigenerational abuse will almost certainly be needed (Hargrave, 1994).

Partners who have experienced long-term relationships and who are now embarking on the Older Adult Lifestyle period because of a dramatic shift in physical, emotional, or mental health on the part of one or both partners find themselves confronted with four clusters of tasks necessary to the continuing prosperity of the marriage (Cole, 1986): first, "realigning the relationship" to ensure a healthy balance of independence, dependence, and interdependence or separateness and togetherness between the couple; second, enhancing interpersonal competencies, such as effective communication, problem-solving skills, and sensitivity to a partner's needs; third, anticipating socialization needs in later life by strengthening support networks outside the marriage and preparing for future periods of older adulthood; and fourth, lifestyle reorganization by adjusting to the particular needs of this particular period. The performance of these tasks may infuse new life into long-standing relationships as well as prepare a marriage for the present and future challenges that confront it.

Relationships Without Partners

For some who find themselves without partners in this period, reinventing the self may also include reinventing family in the form of marriage. Such unions may occur at any age, but the period following the Early Transition provides a common setting for those who have been recently widowed or those individuals who have recently relocated. Since "till death do you part isn't so long when you're in your sixties" (Heilbrun, 1997, p. 109), or seventies, or eighties, the agenda for newly married relationships often contains a sense of urgency and intensity about establishing the new family unit. A danger occurs when new couples withdraw into their own happiness, as if to block out the rest of the world. The need to forge and maintain relationships persists, whether married or single; the reality is that half of those currently united in marriage will be single again during their lifetime. However, the diversity of the older adult population is reflected in the marital data: whereas about 75 percent of men live with their spouses, more than half of women live alone (*Older Americans 2000: Key Indicators of Well Being,* 2000).

Some without partners find that living together as same- or opposite-sex couples provides the companionship and support they seek without the legal and financial ramifications of marriage. In some instances, unrelated older adults live together in a platonic relationship for convenience, support, and companionship; in others, unrelated older adults live together as conjugal partners without benefit of marriage for many of the same reasons. For some older adults, cohabitation is seen less as a prelude to marriage and more as an alternative, meeting needs without the paraphernalia of a formalized relationship. Older persons are discovering that there is more than one way to be family. Recent census data indicate that this group is growing dramatically. The U.S. Census Bureau reports a total of nearly 5 million households consisting of two unrelated persons, 4 percent of whom are headed by a person in the 65 to 74 age group, and 3 percent of whom are in the age group 75 and above (2001a). The Census Bureau's Current Population Survey shows about 203,000 households contain two unrelated adults, a man and a woman, at least one of whom is 65 or older, in either a conjugal relationship or as friends. This number is 60 percent greater than that of 1990 and 71 percent greater than that of 1980 (CBS News, 2002).

The search for companionship, often through dating and sexual liaison, has resulted in contraction of HIV/AIDS derived from infection through sexual contact among the older adult population. Approximately 1.5 percent of AIDS cases through 2001 were reported by persons age 65 and above (Centers for Disease Control and Prevention, 2001a), and the number of cases of both men and women who have contracted AIDS from heterosexual contact has increased (Centers for Disease Control and Prevention, 1998). However, the proportion of the AIDS cases in the population over 50 has remained stable over time, and the death rate from AIDS among persons over 65 actually decreased between the years 1994 and 2000 (Centers for Disease Control and Prevention, 2003).

Among both friends and family, this time is one of building and maintaining community. As the result of changes in situation, relocation, and death, older persons may find themselves virtually alone. So long as they are able, they fend for themselves and assume they are doing okay. But isolation exacts a high price; research provides evidence that lack of daily contact with others may lead to chronic stress and depression, opening the way to illnesses such as heart disease or lowered immune functioning. Isolation is not the same as solitude, just as being alone is not the same as being lonely. Prolonged and persistent isolation has a devastating impact, but, conversely, all need quiet times alone, for meditation and contemplation, for self-renewal and self-discovery.

Being surrounded by those who give and receive love and support, receiving feedback as the self is reinvented, enjoying companionship and stimulation, may be one of the crowning blessings of the older adult years, as reinventing one's self is accompanied by reinventing one's community.

FREEDOM

For some older adults, freedom translates into the ability to maintain control of one's life, to be accountable to and for oneself, and to retain a level of autonomy and independence. The outcome of freedom for this population is dignity, self-respect, self-control, personal initiative, an intensity of purpose, and such other attributes demonstrate that one is responsible for one's life. Dolly caught a sense of this when she said, "The best thing about being my age is, saying what you want to say and doing what you really want to do; and saying 'No, I don't want to do it . . . ,' not having to be coerced into doing things that you'd prefer not to do." To a considerable degree, Dolly was voicing a value of the dominant culture, where freedom translates into autonomy and control.

In this setting, believing that one is in charge of one's life is critical to one's well-being, particularly in the dominant culture. But there are threats that challenge and undermine. Well-meaning family members at a distance or institutions close at hand may take over decision making on the assumption that they can perform functions more efficiently and with less bother. Programs designed to aid older people are often founded on the notion that with age comes inability. Therefore, instead of aiding older people to perform tasks, program personnel may perform services in place of them. The message that this conveys to older adults is that their competence is rapidly decreasing, and their personal ability to plan and implement actions is reduced, reinforcing whatever negative assessments they may have about themselves. Self-respect is hard to maintain when others intervene and assume responsibility under the guise of assistance. Professionals and family members who assist older adults are in particularly advantageous situations to enable older adults in this period to exercise combined freedom and responsibility in setting goals and implementing them.

Signs of loss of control become the harbinger of future devastation. Cracks in the veneer portend potential signs of senility, dependence, and future losses and decline. Barbara Myerhoff (1978) described the symptoms: "A forgotten word, an outburst of temper, a non sequitur, a misplaced object, a lapse of judgment or reasoning were all scrutinized as ominous portents that the process of decay was beginning" (p. 181). Fears may prompt such caution as to immobilize, and, paradoxically, in protecting self-control a person may sacrifice freedom by becoming reclusive or defensive. The loss of control may also result in a person being marginalized—set aside from the mainstream. The larger quality of life suffers in the simple effort to maintain self-respect.

One important consequence of loss of control is the loss of self-esteem, the value a person places on the self. Such a loss in one's estimation of oneself is understandable when one concludes that life and the activities of living are beyond a person's means to control or enact. Notions that life is too complex and that its myriad responsibilities are overwhelming add to the sense of one's diminished self-worth.

In many ethnic traditions, such as African-American, Hispanic, Native American, and immigrant populations, treating the older person as the most respected person in the family is an important value, and with age, respect is accompanied by care. The most respected one has a high level of control, but it is often characterized by a family's care rather than the older adult's autonomy. Freedom is interpreted as freedom from responsibility and initiative. The acculturation into the dominant culture of younger generations of ethnic families suggests that the continuation of an ethic of respectful care may be problematic, as in the case of the Navaho elders who mourned the loss of the "old ways" by their children who had left the reservation to live in the city and who were unavailable to show the parents either respect or care.

Similarly, thoughtful persons of any cultural tradition may discover that a satisfactory alternative is to reduce the scope of their domain to a size in which they are able to be comfortable. Domain may refer to residence, or activities, or any other aspect of their lives. Giving one's options and boundaries a realistic appraisal and reducing one's aspirations to what seems feasible given the circumstances serves to make one's life more manageable. As the result, voluntarily limiting purposes and activities results in an increased level of self-esteem (Huyck & Hoyer, 1982, p. 249).

For some, across all cultural traditions, freedom expands beyond the careful calculation of control designed to maintain autonomy into the confidence to defy expectations of conformity. Although society lacks normative role models for older citizens who have moved past Extended Middle Age, every reader could list examples of the unwritten code in every community, if not in every family, that prescribes older adult behavior. Older adults who fail to "act their age" become newsworthy: octogenarians who run in marathons, graduate from universities, play softball, work full-time, run for public office, hike the Appalachian Trail, provide child care to great-grandchildren, wear miniskirts and bikinis, bike throughout Europe, teach effective farming methods to younger persons, and volunteer for disaster relief teams have been the subject of news coverage, not because of the newsworthiness of the activity itself, but because their behavior deviates from the expectations that these activities will be enjoyed by younger persons. *The New York Times* even printed a rotogravure story on women over 60 who served as models at a Paris fashion show (Thomas, 1995, p. 22).

Sylvia Townsend Warner (Heilbrun, 1997, p. 55) wrote in her diary:

> In the evening, the Amadeus [Quartet] played opus 132; and I danced to the last movement, I rose up and danced, among the cats, and their saucers, and only when I was too far carried away to stop did I realize that I was behaving very oddly for my age— and that perhaps it was the last time I would dance for joy.*

One older person lifted freedom in older adulthood to a new level:

> Freedom to be me, whatever me I have invented, me as I have always wanted to be. The cost of this freedom goes down each year, because each year I have less to lose. I can't lose my job. I can't lose my future. I can afford to take risks that I could never afford to take before. That's freedom.

PURPOSES AND PRIORITIES

A person in the Older Adult Lifestyle period doesn't need reminders of mortality. Bodily aches and malfunctions, the loss of friends, and one's own clock are constant reminders that there is less of life to live. For some, this spells gloom and depression. For others, it calls for intensity of purpose and the setting of priorities. What to do in the time that is left? What are the priorities? What activities fulfill personal ambitions, complete a lifelong agenda, make a great difference in an institution or community, make a difference in the lives of individuals or a group? What shall be the focus of these years?

One should not mistake purpose and focus for busyness. A bumper sticker cautioned, "Look busy. Jesus is coming." The questionable theology of the message belies a covert scheme on the part of many, to the effect that "if only we are preoccupied enough, if we but accumulate enough, the Grim Reaper will mistake us for immortals" (Hull, 2000, p. 124).

In each period of this developmental scheme, the question of meaning and purpose arises. In each, there is the opportunity to iden-

---

*From LETTERS by Sylvia Townsend Warner, published by Chatto & Windus. Reprinted by permission of The Random House Group Ltd.

tify a vocation, to follow a calling. So it is now—but with a twist. Earlier periods have not forced discrimination as this one does. The limitations of time and capacity place a limitation on purpose and priorities, particularly for those who enter this period in their late seventies and beyond. This means that goals must be tailored, aspirations focused, plans designed to fit the time and circumstance.

Those with most difficulty are those who still carry the burden of a broad unfinished agenda. The setting now involves both commitment to a goal and the recognition of its feasibility. Many widows, for example, express dismay that they cannot follow the plan they developed with their husbands, involving travel and other leisure activities based on ample resources. With the husband's death, the plan is no longer feasible, and so trying to follow it brings only disappointment and frustration. Living in the past, while furnishing important memories, both obscures and frustrates the present. But a person who abandons purpose is in danger of losing the self. It is time for a new plan, one that is based in this case on the priorities and interests of a single woman and her resources. Similarly, couples and partners must tailor their purposes to the resources—both financial and physical—available to them.

Priority setting also involves consideration of commitments for the long term, commitments designed to outlast the giver. This may mean planting a tree whose shade and fruit will be enjoyed by the next generation, strengthening an institution whose work will continue long into the future, or endowing a program whose complete fruition will come after the donor is gone. It may mean spending more time with a grandchild, or with other children in the neighborhood. For some, this results in buildings and scholarships named after the donors and plaques in their honor. For others, it means sharing artwork for their children and grandchildren to enjoy, or pieces of furniture used in the family for generations. For one grandmother, it means hand-knitted sweaters for family members, useful gifts certain to outlast her and infuse the future with memories of her life. Family possessions are usually the stuff of which estate sales are made. But they can stand as continuing reminders of prior users, stewards of their care for a time, and of the relationships that surrounded their use. In one family there is a small pump organ, the wedding gift of a great-great-grandfather to his bride, and the center of family singing for generations. Someday it will belong to a new generation to fulfill its time-honored purpose. Possessions may be baggage, but when shared, they become sacraments.

OLD AGE IS NOT FOR SISSIES

This chapter began on a somber note, its thoughts born out of the experience of Early Transition following Extended Middle Age. It ends on a similar note, since this period ends in another transition, one that anticipates a greater diminution of capacity and autonomy. In other words, this extended period of Older Adult Lifestyle is bookended with the experience of loss. Jonathan Hull (2000, p. 296) reminds us that all of our lives "are a struggle between love and loss."

For many, loss is the operative word at this time in older adulthood. The dominant theme is "Everything goes . . ." Parodies describe loss of bodily and mental functions and point to ways life is diminishing with the loss of energy within and the loss of time ahead. The message is filled with all that will be left behind—not only possessions, but friendships, and music, and secret loves and joys. For many, fear of declining health and the prospect of pain and suffering tower over thoughts of the shortness of days.

For some, deeply rooted in the present, love dominates despite the reality of losses. Anticipation of these losses does not necessitate loss of spirit. It may instill the determination to live each day as if it were the most important, as if it were a unique gift, or as if it were the last. Someone aptly described this time as "not for sissies." It calls upon its inhabitants to muster strength, rely on experience, and pull together fortitude in order to share in that triumph of the spirit that allows older persons not only to endure the latter years, but to prevail over the losses that would subvert the purpose, the friendship, and joyous potential of this time of life. Several years ago, when Bob Edwards of National Public Radio's *Morning Edition* asked sports commentator Red Barber what he was doing for Thanksgiving, Barber responded simply, "Bob, when you're 86, every day is Thanksgiving!" Aging is not for sissies; it is for those with indomitable and grateful spirits.

Chapter 6

The Later Transition

When our first parents were driven out of Paradise, according to a *New Yorker* cartoon, Adam is reported to have remarked to Eve, "My dear, we live in an age of transition." This apocryphal anecdote speaks to much of aging and, indeed, much of life—one transition after another. Although change is often discomforting, if not threatening, the Later Transition may test the ability to accommodate change as has no other period. It tests at many levels: it tests egos, it tests faith and conviction, it tries resolve and determination, and it defies many coping strategies. It tests resolve to prevail with flexibility and imagination over expected and unexpected obstacles in the experience of frailty, illness, and disability. It challenges the ability to grow from the experience.

The Later Transition refers to a transition, usually of one year or less, from independence to dependence. The actual transition may take place in the brief time that marks the tipping point between older adults' ability to care for themselves and the admission that they can no longer make it on their own.

A great many of the broad negative images surrounding older adulthood, to say nothing of personal fears about late life, are concentrated in this transition. In a national survey identifying the greatest worries people have about growing older, respondents were most concerned about becoming a financial burden to their children, getting a life-threatening disease, ending up in a nursing home, and losing their attractiveness—the very eventualities that may occur during this period (Perry, 2001). The notion of dependence may carry its own negative connotations, creating visions of a useless, unwanted burden,

A Journey Called Aging: Challenges and Opportunities in Older Adulthood
© 2007 by The Haworth Press, Taylor & Francis Group. All rights reserved.
doi:10.1300/5915_07

although for some it will also have the positive dimensions of freedom from responsibility and ready access to care.

The landmark that distinguishes the Later Transition is the inability to live independently and includes such related losses as health, mobility, and autonomy. There have been many losses in older adulthood, beginning with retiring, that may have included loss of the identity employment provided, loss of income, loss of a spouse, and loss of close friends. If one widens the view, one is faced with a giant tapestry of loss, where current losses blend into every deprivation experienced since middle age, giving the feeling that all the losses of a lifetime are piling up and threatening to crush one's very self. Concerns expand to include fear of abandonment, of no longer belonging, and of being forgotten. One grieves for losses in the past and the present, anticipating a future where the loss will be final and complete.

As the journey of life moves forward at its own pace, it develops a sense of transiency and impermanence, a sense described by Benjamin Franklin when he said, "I still exist, and still enjoy some pleasures in that existence. . . . Yet I feel the infirmities of age come on so fast, and the building to need so many repairs, that in a little time the owner will find it cheaper to pull it down and build a new one" (Boyd, 2001, p. x). During this period, many of a person's hopes about older adulthood are shown to be illusions. Opportunities for enrichment and fulfillment are replaced with the consuming struggle to maintain health and comfort. For many, well-being is challenged by the onset of frailty, debility, and dementia. That the age group over 85 is the most rapidly growing segment of the population is due in large part to medical advances that have improved health status earlier in life and have brought large numbers of older adults to this stage. Ironically, during the later transition medical miracles seem to have run their course, offering a more limited hope of complete recovery from the maladies and diseases that afflict many older persons.

Many older persons have developed a personal vision of the circumstances under which they would like to meet death. A common denominator of most such images is that death comes suddenly in the midst of health. One person said he would like to take a walk in the park, come home, lie down to rest, and be gone. Many hope that it will happen as they sleep, after an evening of conversation with good friends, or a time of making love, or similar favorite activities. The

Later Transition disabuses those holding to these idyllic visions of death with the clear warning that it will likely not be so easy. This period for many seems to be the transition between life and death writ large.

THE ROLE OF PROFESSIONALS AND SUPPORT PERSONS

Decreased independence combined with increasing diminishment resulting from accumulated losses frames the need of older adults in the Later Transition for professional assistance as well as the support of family and friends. While many of the helping roles required at this time are similar to those required in earlier periods, their importance now is amplified by the onset of greater dependence that may require a greater initiative and a broader understanding on the part of professionals and others. Chronic and lingering issues that were annoyances, but that had not risen to the level of irritants, may now have become major concerns requiring immediate resolution. Earlier decisions about housing and care, for example, are inevitably revisited even though the momentum involved in those decisions may be difficult to redirect.

At the same time, older adults directly involved in the transition often resist the changes that this transition will introduce and work to postpone it as long as possible. Professionals and other helpers are sometimes placed in the role of catalysts for change, bringing expertise and influence to bear in such a way as to resolve an untenable situation. In some instances, recalcitrance to change in spite of evident dependency will challenge caregivers and supporters alike.

It is incumbent upon all who work with older persons to understand the nature of the support that is available. Common expectations within the dominant culture anticipate that the principal members of a support network will most likely consist of spouses and lineal descendants if they exist. Less likely will siblings be involved, and still less likely will the children of siblings or nonrelatives provide support. By contrast, patterns of support in the African-American community include vital roles for spouses, children, siblings, adult grandchildren, and adult nieces or nephews, depending on availability. According to Luckey (1994), second and third generation kin are likely to be better educated and be able to connect to the formal system of care more knowledgeably than their older kin. To summarize Luckey's (1994) illustration,

> a 76-year-old single, African American woman with a seventh-grade education was unable to make financial ends meet when she could no longer work at her two part-time domestic jobs. Her siblings were aware of her financial difficulties. She was a proud, self-reliant woman and was adamant about not going on welfare. Her sister told the sister's daughter, a 32-year-old-college graduate, about the situation. The niece contacted several people in her network of colleagues and friends to obtain information about possible assistance for her aunt. She called a Social Security office for information about Supplemental Security Income, then shared this information with her mother and aunt, encouraging her aunt to apply. (p. 83)

Informal support networks that include siblings and extend to several generations may provide a challenge to professionals who fail to understand and make use of the resources that an extended family has available. They may also present a problem to institutions and programs in which policies that govern information sharing fail to accommodate the involvement of a broad network consisting of various relatives and friends.

At the same time, older members of all cultural groups may experience a decrease in the availability of family support. Decreasing family size, increasing mobility of family members, employment of both women and men outside the home, and acculturation of minorities all contribute to the diminishment of extensive support networks, increasing the roles that professionals may be expected to assume. Provision of care is exacerbated among some cultural groups by high expectations that care will be provided by family members and by the traditionally limited use of extended-care facilities. For example, estimates place utilization of nursing homes by African Americans at between one-half and three-quarters of that of whites (Belgrave, Wykle, & Choi, 1993).

Another important function of those who work with persons engaged in this transition is to advocate for adequate care in the health care, social service, and mental health communities. Accusations of ageism still persist in discussions of the care of older adults, in some cases because the professionals who treat them lack training in gerontology or geriatrics. The Alliance of Aging Research (2003) reported the following: (1) older people are often denied the kind of preventive care routinely provided to others; (2) older people are less likely to be screened for life-threatening diseases; (3) proven medical interventions for older people are often ignored, leading to inappropriate or incomplete treatment; and (4) older people are consistently under represented in—or even excluded from—clinical trials.

At a hearing conducted by the U.S. Senate Special Committee on Aging, the Assistant Secretary for Aging of the U.S. Department of Health and Human Services (Carbonell, 2003) projected that the growth of older adults, particularly in the 85 plus age group, will likely exceed the supply of long-term care workers. Positively, professionals may also play a role in helping develop adequate strategies for care that take into account both personal financial resources and availability of persons to serve as caregivers.

In addition to advocating for the best health care available, professionals must recognize that many older persons, especially those from ethnic and immigrant populations, have a history of reliance on alternative healing strategies born of their respective cultural traditions. The use of faith healing, *curanderismo,* among Hispanics, the Native American use of traditional Indian medicines for the treatment of chronic illness, the Chinese American use of acupuncture and acupressure, the widespread use of herbal and natural substances as well as prayer and spiritual practices are examples. Ethnicity determines attitudes, values, and expectations of old age and extends to beliefs about health and healing as well.

Particular professionals may become dispassionately involved in the discussion of a range of ethical issues, from the use of the children's inheritance for long-term care of a frail parent to the morality of certain medical interventions to the rights of individuals to determine when to "pull the plug."

Professionals and other support persons may be expected to look beyond their individual specialties and areas of expertise to a holistic view of the person. This view requires a sensitivity not only to particular diagnoses of physical, mental, or emotional ills, but also to the overriding personal concerns of the individual. Persons engaged in this transition may need help interpreting their situation, answering the question "What is happening to me?," maintaining contact with the outside world beyond immediate caregivers, understanding the nature of the contribution they are able to make to their families and friends despite their dependency, and knowing when to hold on and when to let go of any number of issues and items. It may also involve helping persons distinguish between what is "normal aging" and what are diseases that may be handled through medication and therapy, and for which there may be some resolution. Persons who combine some level of objectivity with the subjectivity of sensitive care are often able to broaden horizons, help persons reflect constructively and creatively on their own state of affairs, and encourage people to help manage their own situations and to maintain or recapture a level of emotional health and resiliency following illness or loss.

BEGINNING THE JOURNEY

How do people get to this transition? Where does the Later Transition begin? As with all life stages, there is no single route. Verbrugge and Jette (1994) have described this transition from activity to disability, beginning with a particular pathology that gives rise to a bodily impairment, which in turn decreases the ability to function, finally resulting in limits on the conduct of daily life and social roles. Early signs may appear when a person experiences frequent falls, or blackouts, or a person's vision no longer allows operation of an automobile, or when painful joints inhibit virtually all movement, or when persons no longer have the energy to care for themselves or their immediate living quarters. The transition unfolds as care begins at a minimal level—perhaps with regular phone calls or visits to make certain that the person's needs are being met—and gradually increases over time to the point where regular support services are required to assist the person in the home. It may conclude at the point where the needs for assistance can no longer be met in the home without a fairly intensive level of care or where full-time assisted care, either from professional or family caregivers, may be necessary.

Sudden Transitions

For some it comes more swiftly in the middle of the Older Adult Lifestyle period, as an accident or illness forces this dramatic change. One ex-farmer described how his children had moved him from his hundred-acre farm to an extended-care facility: "The thing is when you get my age you sometimes pass out, or you fall and you get hurt easily . . . out in the sticks where there's no one around . . . their reasoning was good." Others are forced into the Later Transition as the result of a devastating accident or illness from which there is no recovery. In the early months of her retirement, an active friend broke her hip in a fall. Her severe osteoporosis had hitherto gone undiagnosed, and now she faced years in which she would have limited mobility and limited ability to care for herself.

A few have fast-forwarded into this period from middle age. A house painter in his sixties, bragging that he would never retire, fell from a scaffold, broke his back, and required care all of his remaining days.

For some, the transition happens abruptly when, after a hospitalization for an illness, they find themselves not strong enough to go back home without daily nursing care, and a nursing home is the only option. This is a particularly difficult journey when the person relies on Medicaid to pay for the nursing home. The first bed that comes available may not be at all close to home or to those most likely to provide support.

And for a few, the transition seems without any redeeming qualities or signs of hope whatever and forces the ultimate alternative. Suicide rates in the United States are highest among persons aged 65 and older. Although this age group accounts for 13 percent of the population, it has accounted for 18 percent of all suicide deaths. The highest suicide rates in the country in 2000 were among white men over 85, with a rate of 59 per 100,000 population, more than five times the national average rate of 10.6 per 100,000 population (National Institute of Mental Health, 2003). Within the over 65 age group, suicide rates increase with age. Rates are higher for males, for those divorced or widowed, and are lower for Hispanics and blacks (U.S. Department of Health and Human Services, n.d.; Hoyert, Arias, Smith, Murphy, & Kochanek, 2001, Tables 9, 10, 14).

Planned Transitions

For most persons, however, this transition comes gradually after a long and healthy older adulthood when, not surprisingly, in their seventies, eighties, or nineties, their bodies finally succumb to frailty and they are no longer able to care for themselves. Frailty is popularly regarded as consisting of some combination of muscular weakness, mental or emotional diminishment, decline in activity, fatigue, an uncertain gait, and weight loss. Frailty may be physical, mental, or emotional, or all three. Judge Oliver Wendell Holmes Jr. used a metaphor not unlike that of Benjamin Franklin quoted earlier, in which he combines the realism of frailty, an underlying sense of integrity, and a good dose of humor. When he was asked at age 92 "And how is Oliver Wendell Holmes today?" he replied:

> Oliver Wendell Holmes is well, quite well, I thank you, but the house in which he lives at present is becoming quite dilapidated. It is tottering upon its foundation. Time and the seasons have nearly destroyed it. Its roof is pretty well worn out. Its walls are much shattered and it trembles with every wind. The old tenement is becoming almost uninhabitable, and I think Oliver Wendell Holmes will have to move out soon. But he himself is well, quite well. (*Johns Hopkins Magazine,* September 1993, p. 28)

Advance planning goes far in contributing to the successful completion of the transition. With proper preparation, maximum use may be made of both financial and personal resources, providing the older adult with some level of involvement in decisions that determine future care, and allowing an opportunity to weigh options and research possibilities.

While planning is important for all, those with limited resources may have particular difficulty in maximizing their impact by a careful balancing of demands with resources. Recent research on financial literacy and planning and their implications for retirement well-being showed that overall "fewer than one-fifth of the respondents believed they engaged in successful retirement planning" (Lusardi & Mitchell, 2005, p. 3). The research further indicated that women, minorities, and those without a college degree were particularly at risk.

For example, for African Americans and Latinos in inner cities, most of whom have put in full working lives, the picture may not be so sanguine. Katherine Newman (2003) describes their experience:

> Now that these middle-aged and elderly residents of our inner cities are approaching the age when they need to rely on the kindness and support of those adult children, reliable relatives may be in short supply. At the same time, the need is great and often arrives early in the lives of inner-city dwellers, who tend to develop chronic health problems earlier than the norm. (pp. 3-4)

Although many ethnic families take pride in providing care for elderly relatives, their ability to do so may be diminishing. Placing an older family member in a care institution may not be so stigmatizing as it once was. Groger and others report that "there exists a cultural lag between the ideals of filial obligation, or the culture of caring, and the material conditions which make it increasingly more difficult to attain the ideal" (Groger, Mayberry, Straker, & Mehdizadeh, 1997, p. 4).

In fact, an increasing number of long-term care facilities are developing programs and facilities that cater to the language and the diet of older members of particular ethnic groups. For example, a Chicago nursing home serves Chinese-speaking residents on one floor and Spanish-speaking residents on another. According to Belgrave and others (1993), the proportion of African Americans to whites in long-term care facilities has increased steadily over the past four decades, from 37 percent in 1963 to 65 percent in 1989. African Americans tend to reside in nursing homes and smaller residential-care/assisted-living facilities that serve predominantly African Americans (Howard et al., 2002). And Groger (1997) notes that in her Ohio-based study, African-American elders are more likely than their white counterparts to go to a nursing home.

TIMING THE TRANSITION

Quite often this transition is postponed as long as possible—and longer than should be. Sophie Ann went twice a week to care for her mother who simply refused to "be put in an old age home." Her mother's condition deteriorated quite quickly, yet she refused to give up her driver's license. For her, the only thing that would tip the balance was the almost-inevitable automobile accident.

The timing of the move to accept help often seems poor. People try to hold on too long. One woman said, "As long as I can still drive I am not going to go into a retirement community." But her ability to make that transition when she can no longer drive (and by implication has depleted health resources and energy) is jeopardized by leaving the transition so late.

Contrast this approach with that of one retired woman. In a statement circulated among members of her family and made an official document in her advance directives, she articulated her desire that when the need for care arises, she be cared for in her home as long as possible. She then lists the circumstances under which she desires to be moved to a community-based assisted-living facility, and the circumstances under which she desires to be moved to a nursing home. This provides both family members and health care professionals with clear information about her preferences, stated at a time when she is able to make decisions about her future. And while she may not always be able to be active in choosing care facilities, she may be confident that the choices others make in her behalf will be in accord with her desires. When a person is no longer able to make decisions about future care, either someone else will make those decisions, or they will be made by default. In anticipation of that time, it is advisable for persons to specify in writing the nature of care they wish to receive, the kind of setting in which they wish to receive it, and the names of persons who are empowered to make these decisions for them. The importance of advanced directives notwithstanding, there is no substitute for familiarity with a lifetime of choices and articulated desires, in which case family members are able to predict patient preferences among health care alternatives.

Sometimes the person who is in the midst of this uncertainty needs help in coming to an appropriate decision. Senator Jean Carnahan (2002) tells this remarkable story of her father's Later Transition:

> After my mother passed away, it was clear to me that my father would be better off in my home. The problem was I lived in Missouri, and he lived in the Washington area all his life. He was asthmatic and diabetic and subject to insulin reactions. He needed

reliable care to make sure he ate properly and exercised regularly. Most of all, he needed the love and support of his family.

While I recognized that he should move in with me, this was not clear to him at all. In fact, it was a real test of my powers of persuasion. I gave him all the logical reasons why he should come home with me. Although he listened, he was not convinced. Finally, in one final desperate appeal, I took his hand and said this to my father: "Remember what you hear in church on Sunday morning? That sometimes you need to make a decision based on faith. This is one of those times. You need to believe that this is going to work."

There was a pause. He replied to me—"Where's my suitcase?" (p. 2)

Not all such stories have happy endings. The issue of when to accept the reality of loss and reorient one's life is crucial. Some will try to hold on to the very last, using up every bit of their energy and resources to stay in their own homes. Older adults with families at a distance are usually reluctant to exchange familiar surroundings and a possible network of friends for the security that comes from living near their children. Friends or family who have been called in to help at the last minute are often appalled at the squalor and filth people endure rather than accept help or move to a care facility. But this is understandable for people who grew up in an era that took great pride in self-sufficiency, or whose only knowledge of care facilities is a memory of the old-age home on the edge of town overlooking the cemetery. Further, people get into a sort of downward spiral, involving increased immobility, poor nutrition, out-of-date or poorly monitored medications, and possibly the burden of caring for a sick spouse. Escape from such a spiral requires sufficient resources and energy to initiate change, but resources and energy are precisely what are lacking.

Some make a move voluntarily and of their own initiative while they still have some reserve strength to make a new start. Nathan and Lillian just moved from their downtown apartment, chosen years ago because it was close to all of the places they enjoyed, to an extended-care facility. They are both still in comparatively good health for their upper eighties but recognize that the time is fast approaching when assisted-living supports will not only be welcome, but necessary. Sam held out as long as could, but finally he was persuaded by his son to move into the spare bedroom for the winter. His house will still be there, and should this not work to his satisfaction, he can move back home. And Evie—never married with no close family left—is challenged not only to plot her next steps, but to formalize what has been a very informal network of friends and fellow church members, and to empower certain persons in that network to make decisions on her behalf when she is no longer able to do so. Troll and others point out that during the latter years, older people may seek to renew family loyalties and relationships, and those who have never married or are without children tend to maintain closer relationships with siblings (Troll, Miller, & Atchley, 1979, p. 123).

Accepting help, even in a relationship of dependency, can be an effective strategy for avoiding overtaxing or even depleting one's mental, social, and motivational resources. Some people get new leases on life when they accept care. Finally, they don't have to "do it all." Perhaps for the first time in months or years they don't have to expend a dysfunctionally high level of energy on everyday tasks (Baltes & Baltes, 1990, p. 20). But, admittedly, there is a fine line between "just manageable difficulty" and a dysfunctionally high use of reserves in an effort to avoid dependency.

Giving help as a caregiver may also mean different things to different persons. For some, it may be viewed as a kind of vocation, a service to which one now devotes one's life. For others, it may range from an obligation demonstrating faithfulness to one demonstrating duty. And for still others, the responsibilities of caregiving may be more demanding, physically, mentally, and emotionally, than they have the capability to fulfill.

THE JOURNEY TO CARE

To a considerable degree, social support, personal environment, financial resources, physical capacities, cultural traditions, and earlier planning establish parameters for this transition. Available skills and resources frequently determine whether the outcome will be positive or negative (Walker et al., 2001, p. 10). Frequently cited sources of disadvantage deriving from gender, race, and ethnicity, lack of pension or other income, and disability or chronic ill health often correlate with meager financial resources that limit one's options and opportunities, perhaps restricting one to assistance from public agencies and programs. Conversely, unlimited financial resources clearly allow for private, skilled care of the highest quality available at whatever location and for whatever length of time desired. Most older adults fall somewhere between unlimited and meager resources. They must make careful choices in order to have adequate care available in the event it is needed.

Important considerations include whether one makes this journey alone or with a spouse or partner, whether one has close friends or a community of support, whether there are relatives close at hand, whether there is someone else to share the decision making or provide minimal levels of care, and whether there is someone else to share the responsibility for daily living tasks. Having support may involve emotional and instrumental as well as financial support. Furthermore, having positive social relationships with others may result in enhanced emotional well-being (dealing with stress, irritation, disappointment, etc.) as well as physical well-being (lower blood pressure) (Ong & Allaire, 2005, p. 476). As many older persons endeavor to stay in their own homes longer, programs that serve older adults in their homes, such as home-delivered meals or daily checks to provide a safety network, also provide crucial social contact.

The demographics indicate after age 75, over one-half of all women live alone. After age 75, 23 percent of men and 60 percent of women are widowed. An additional 8 percent of men and 8.4 percent of women are divorced or never married (U.S. Census Bureau, 2001b). After age 85, no more than 20 percent live with a partner (Walker et al., 2001, p. 235). In African-American and Hispanic populations, older women are less likely to live with a spouse and more likely to live with relatives when they are older (Carstensen, 2001, p. 267). In instances where marital partners live together, women are more likely than their husbands to be caregivers (Carstensen, 2001, p. 267). Women are also more likely to be widowed and poor than men and, as they live longer than men, are more likely to suffer from chronic conditions that reduce their ability to carry out the activities of daily living (Heidrich, 1993).

These demographics confirm the view seen in earlier stages: gender, resources, and marital status continue to refute the notion that "one size fits all." Although none of these variables wards off the transition, they do establish significant parameters for the journey and help to influence both the affirming and the shadow dimensions of care.

Good News and Bad

Whether begun swiftly or gradually, involuntarily or with careful planning, the journey to care is marked by considerable ambiguity. Among persons in the dominant culture, although care is needed, care is resisted. Independence is no longer an option; dependency grates against a lifetime of initiative. Control is proving difficult; giving up control to another runs counter to a lifetime of seizing control and protecting it. Tracy Kidder (1993) articulates the dilemma and solution of a pair of nursing-home residents: "He and Lou could not control most of the substance of their life in here, but they had imposed a style on it" (p. 74). In some circles, "I don't want to be a burden to my children" is a mantra of the continuing effort to be independent. However, desire for independence in the face of the need for support has been shown to be strongly impacted by individual and gender-based propensities: for example, men with a high desire to be independent responded negatively to receiving support from their social network, whereas women's outcomes were generally unaffected by their desires for independence or dependence, suggesting that individual and gender-based considerations be taken into account when generalizing about the unequivocal desire for independence (Nagurney, Reich, & Newsom, 2004, p. 215).

The good news about increased levels of care begins with the increasing numbers of options available, from home care to care in a wide variety of institutional settings. The transition usually puts one in closer contact with regular medical attention, something that may have been neglected or overlooked during the preceding older adult years. In many instances it also restores or revitalizes family and social networks that may have lain dormant over a number of years. Increased care also tends to increase well-being. According to George Vaillant's (2002) book *Aging Well*, "the majority of older people, without brain disease, maintain a sense of modest well-being until the final months before they die" (p. 5).

In many minority traditions, however, the culture of aging de-emphasizes autonomy in favor of strong family or ethnic community support and values. For example, among black Americans over the age of 85, a high level of contentment with their lives was associated with (1) social integration into their family, the black church, and the black community; (2) cultural values and beliefs that celebrate old age and create an aura of survivorship; and (3) a sense of well-being based on a comparison of hardships experienced in the past with their current lives (Johnson, 1995, p. 231).

Individuals in a study of whites aged 85 and above were found to have experienced enhanced well-being despite social and physical losses. Johnson and Barer (1997) called them survivors because they interpret their life experiences as beneficial and, instead of falling into depression, think of themselves in ways appropriate to their circumstances, narrowing the focus and range of their activities, and carefully scheduling time to maximize their energy and capabilities. In rethinking their situations, new ideas about autonomy and independence emerge to welcome help from others on whom they now depend.

Although it may be good news to have lived long enough to reach this stage of life, not all would agree that living this long really is preferable to the alternative. Many, given a choice, would elect not to live to this stage. As one diagnosed with a terminal disease recently confided to his doctor, "I am not afraid to die. But I am afraid to suffer." Others don't want their families to see them suffering or want their families to suffer because of them. Good news notwithstanding, the Later Transition continues the journey of change, and baggage for it combines themes of dread, dependency, pain, care, and relief. It is both a blessing and a curse.

Anticipating the Journey

In anticipation of Later Transition, is there any "useful homework"? Most certainly! Research studies confirm that individuals who have choices and make decisions regarding their present and future live better and longer, and exhibit a higher level of well-being and satisfaction. Those who lack choices or autonomy suffer adverse effects, such as lower life satisfaction, lack of a sense of well-being, and emotional and physical instability. Those who believe that they are in charge of their lives and can influence what happens to them have a higher level of self-esteem and self-worth (Rowe & Kahn, 1987).

Among a sample of Mexican Americans, researchers confirmed that good psychological health has protective benefits against poor health outcomes. They found that among those who had a positive attitude toward life, the chances of becoming frail were significantly lower. The results suggest that having a positive attitude toward life may have a number of beneficial health outcomes, including greater functional independence, mobility, and survival (Ostir, Ottenbacher, & Markides, 2004, p. 402). Conversely, in this correlational study, one might argue that those who look optimistically toward the future are more likely to remain physically and socially active.

Lillian E. Troll (2002), a former professor at Rutgers University and current adjunct professor at the University of California, epitomizes the relationship between choices and a strong sense of self:

> Is it a good idea to live alone in old age? Well, it all depends . . . I have lived alone for many years. But I lived with others in the past, too, and can say that I liked living with others but right now I love living alone.
>
> Were I to feel lonely or helpless or were I in need of care, I could change my mind. It is partly a matter of control: control over my territory. It is partly a matter of companionship and sociability: access to other people when I want them. It is partly a matter of independence, which is part of control. It certainly depends on my ability to function—how much help I need to do what I want to do. (p. 9)

But not all plan or even anticipate the need to plan and to be in control. For some, cultural traditions already provide a template for this period, should they choose to follow it. The experience of stability dissolving into change is part of the fabric of life. The organization of this book makes explicit a flow in which the stability of a career transitions into retiring, Extended Middle Age dissolves into the Early Transition, and the Older Adult Lifestyle ends in the move from autonomy to dependency. Yet for all its predictability, awareness of the process does not guarantee adequate personal planning for the transition into dependency or the time of dependency itself. Not all can envision themselves at this stage. Many are genuinely surprised to have lived so long that the later transition becomes an issue. This vignette is part of a story by Edna Ferber, "Old Man Minick":

> There was little or no talk of death between [them]. But as always, between husband and wife, it was understood wordlessly (and without reason) that old man Minick would go first. Not that either of them had the slightest intention of going. . . . Then came the day when Ma Minick went downtown to see Matthews about that pain right here and came home looking shriveled, talking shrilly about nothing, and evading Pa's eyes. Followed months that were just a jumble of agony, X-rays, hope, despair, morphia, nothingness.
>
> After it was all over: "But I was going first," old man Minick said, dazedly. (Cited in Merriam, 1983, p. 89)

Sufficient information is available about the possibility and the experience of this transition as to warrant serious planning. MacBean and Simmons (2006) identify three questions that are integral to preparing for a time of frailty: (1) Where will you live? (2) How will you pay for it? and (3) How will you live? They call this process "frailty planning." "Where will you live?" explores strategic options of locations and types of facilities, with their dreams, pros, and cons. "How will you pay for it?" examines issues of financial security throughout aging, including frailty. "How will you live?" explores the profound impact of character on thriving in body, mind, heart, and soul through to the end of life, even in a period of dependency and care.

Gene Cohen suggests the development of a "social portfolio" in which assets are diversified, a safety net is in place, and the investment begins as early as possible. His plan directs persons to broaden their interests and relationships and to "cultivate a healthy range of interests that include group and individual activities that require high energy/high mobility as well as low energy/low mobility" ("Seven 'Secrets' to Healthy Aging," 1999), and to take these steps immediately in order to prepare for life as one ages. This is sound advice, although it does not take away the effect of happenstance and uncontrollable realities.

Choosing Where to Live

Unplanned transitions are more difficult to negotiate than those that have been anticipated and for which preparation has been made. This is particularly true in the Later Transition.

Options for care are directly linked to choices about the "best" place to live. Simmons and MacBean (2006) group choices into five categories: (1) staying in one's home and getting needed services there; (2) living with an adult family member, and counting on that person's kindness and purchased services for help; (3) living in a continuing-care retirement community that provides all services from independent living through health care; (4) living communally with friends, sharing duties and resources; and (5) moving as needed (and as late as possible) to increasingly more complex levels of care—for example, from home to assisted living, and then to a nursing home. Within each of these possible choices there are a variety of options for care and support. While it is not the task of this book to discuss them in detail, the reader who wishes to be prepared for the uncertain journey would do well to study local options and opportunities for care, recognizing that any decline in function increases dependency on one's environment and makes one more susceptible to negative outcomes resulting from living in an inappropriate environment (Krout & Wethington, 2003, p. 5). Research findings suggest that

[a]lthough those who relocated experienced declines in functional health, they reported significantly greater well-being, measured as psychological morale and life satisfaction, than did those who remained in the community. Housing in senior residences appeared to buffer individuals against some of the negative effects of health decline, with psychological well-being and social involvement remaining at relatively favorable levels. (Boyce, Wethington, & Moen, 2003, p. 178)

Some people begin their preparations in Extended Middle Age. One couple has decided that their ranch-style home in a beautiful surrounding is an ideal setting for their latter years. What could they do now to make certain it is suitable when the time comes? Their list includes wider doors, new lighting, laundry facilities on the main floor, and a bath that would accommodate someone using a wheelchair. Others visit open houses at new retirement villages, senior apartments, assisted-living facilities, continuing-care communities, and similar venues in order to acquaint themselves with both the possibilities and the costs. Plans can then be made without the pressure of immediate need. Shopping ahead of need is well-founded advice.

Often the development of an informal plan for next steps expands to include other necessary components, such as the development of advanced directives for health care, the disposition of possessions, the plan for the celebration of one's life. For Marge, home assistance is already a fact. And at some point, it will become inadequate and give way to a move to an assisted-living facility.

> It was Thanksgiving, and she invited her three kids and any available grandchildren to her townhouse to celebrate the holiday. But she had more in mind: it was a time when she gave some favorite family items—some furniture, some jewelry, some antiques, and other special pieces—to the next generation. She didn't give away everything, but the process of passing down was well initiated. They also toured some assisted-living facilities in the surrounding community. Then she began discussing plans for her memorial service—where it would be held, who would participate, and how it would be conducted. Her children became participants in the planning, and by their involvement signed on to her wishes. With that she planned the celebration in greater detail, and even invited those from outside the family whom she wished to participate in a memorial event sometime in the future. Home care continued for four years, until plans for moving to assisted living were implemented.

Although extended-care facilities may seem unattractive when compared with one's own home, advocates note that one important element in a retirement community is "community," and the combination of persons and services that overcome loneliness, physical isolation, and burdensome responsibilities for care can give one a new lease on life.

In contrast to such facilities, others expect their adult children to care for them; it is part of their life experience, their family culture, and it seems eminently right. In an earlier era when the multigenerational family was the norm, the Later Transition would have occurred entirely within the home, as certain female family members would have assumed responsibility for caring for a frail elderly relative. In fact, many of today's septuagenarians and octogenarians developed their earliest views of older adulthood while growing up in homes where families—usually a mother whose work was primarily at home (or on the home farm)—cared for older relatives. This has left many of today's older adults with a strong sense of the fundamental rightness of being cared for at home by a daughter, or strong memories of the delight a grandmother or older aunt took in seeing them every day after school, or—for some—darker memories of disability or illness that accompanied age. Decisions about where care may be available depend on family willingness, cultural traditions, resource availability, as well as other factors.

By planning ahead for the eventuality of care—the "frailty planning" mentioned earlier—one is able to set directions and parameters for care. Nevertheless, others will be living with another set of options. They will have done nothing, waiting to see if they live long enough to need such care. In this case, circumstances will dictate from a list of those possibilities that are available at the time of need.

Options for Care

The care industry is big business and getting bigger. For example, a decade ago, assisted-living facilities were almost unknown. Now there are thousands of such facilities offering a variety of levels of assistance with the needs of people at various levels of frailty. Hospitals, residential retirement communities, and home care health agencies offer services-for-fee for people who want to stay in their own homes or in the home of a relative. Because of the development of a range of increasing options for care, nursing homes are being used mainly for rehabilitation and for long-term care, often for persons with dementia. Responding to the need for information about options for care, a new program that makes available vast amounts of data on patients in every nursing home in the country can be viewed on the Medicare program's Web site at http://www.medicare.gov (U.S. Department of Health and Human Services, n.d.).

In some areas, the care industry is about the business of customizing its services to respond to the diverse interests of new generations of potential residents. In an issue of *Road and Track,* the members of a "garage band" who were approaching 50 dreamed about an "old people's home" where they would be able to bring their amps and drums and guitars as well as their wrenches. It could even have garage bays for working on old cars—preferable to playing checkers, they believed (Egan, 1996, p. 32). These fantasies may seem far-fetched, but facilities are recognizing that programs at care facilities need to respond to a broad range of interests and levels of functionality. Accommodations are beginning to reflect more varied and active lifestyles, even in environments designed for care.

Planning for a time of dependency and care takes advantage of opportunities but requires levels of information that may not be readily available without help. Constance Hale (2000, p. 136) identifies these experts to rely on when the time comes: (1) the information specialist at the local Area Agency on Aging; (2) a private geriatric care manager who can assist with complex arrangements, especially if family members live in locations distant from the person requiring care; (3) a hospital discharge planner who can help arrange placements in rehabilitation centers, nursing homes, or make arrangements for home care; (4) a family therapist who can aid in the resolution of conflict related to patient care within the family; (5) an elder law attorney to help with estate planning as well as advance directives such as living wills, health care power of attorney, and durable power of attorney; and (6) a certified financial planner to manage assets and plan financing for care needs.

There are also online resources for planning and for responding to the vagaries of this Later Transition. A model of these online resources is www.seniornavigator.com for the State of Virginia (Senior Navigator, n.d.). Along with a wealth of up-to-date information on every aspect of growing old, one feature stands out: any resource can be located by city, town, or zip code.

No matter in which environment one chooses to receive care, factors such as the adequacy of the facility and equipment, the competency of care, and the feasibility of cost require careful consideration. Of equal importance are less tangible elements such as opportunities for socialization, care for mental as well as physical health, social activities appropriate to one's level of well-being, and activities designed to provide intellectual stimulation. Even the frail elderly benefit both physically and mentally from physical exercise as diverse as chair aerobics and strength training.

Decisions made in Later Transition that involve leaving one's own home can be difficult to reverse. The decision to stay in one's home or that of a relative may seem less "perpetual," but it too will have some momentum that will be difficult to alter. Always, the person who is in Later Transition and those helping with decisions need to be attentive to the potentially traumatic nature of this transition. At the same time, most participants have a lifetime of well-honed coping skills and varying levels of resilience. Robert Kastenbaum (1993) describes them as having a self-protective level of encrustation that resists actual and perceived threats (p. 174). Some have suggested that this resilience results from the ability of older persons to limit the number of things that concern them; others have documented the tendency of older people to regulate their emotions by maintaining positive feelings through the recall of fewer negative images (Charles, Mather, & Carstensen, 2003). These possible explanations combined with a perception of the present as a precursor to fulfillment, growth, or just a time relieved of suffering or responsibility make the transition less an ending and more a gateway to whatever future may be envisioned.

Ruth Howard Gray's (1986) book *Survival of the Spirit: My Detour In and Out of a Retirement Home* sums up some of the challenge as she presents excerpts from a diary written in her eighty-fifth year. They reveal a woman's struggle to maintain her individuality and personhood in a retirement home in the face of inflexible and insensitive administrators. The author and her peers emerge as positive, creative, but embattled people. Although their Later Transition has very dark, unredeemed moments, one ends the book with a sense of hope, which is how this transition, at its best, concludes. They do survive and prevail, modeling the journey for all who find themselves on this pathway.

Chapter 7

While the Light Lasts

In his poem "Ithaka," C. P. Cavafy (1995) draws a picture that can be seen as a metaphor for the journey to and arrival at the final stable period of life, "While the light lasts":

Hope the voyage is a long one.
May there be many a summer morning when,
with what pleasure, what joy,
you come into harbors seen for the first time;
may you stop at Phoenician trading stations
to buy fine things, mother of pearl and coral, amber and ebony,
sensual perfume of every kind—
as may you visit many Egyptian cities
to gather stores of knowledge from their scholars.

Keep Ithaka always in your mind.
Arriving there is what you are destined for.
But do not hurry the journey at all.
Better if it lasts for years,
so you are old by the time you reach the island,
wealthy with all you have gained on the way,
not expecting Ithaka to make you rich.

Ithaka gave you the marvelous journey.
Without her you would not have set it out.
She has nothing left to give you now.

A Journey Called Aging: Challenges and Opportunities in Older Adulthood
© 2007 by The Haworth Press, Taylor & Francis Group. All rights reserved.
doi:10.1300/5915_08

And if you find her poor, Ithaka won't have fooled you.
Wise as you will have become, so full of experience,
you will have understood by then what these Ithakas mean.*
(p. 25)

Whatever its integrity, distinctiveness, and stark boundaries, this period of life can only be understood in the context of a whole life, at the end of which "you are old, wealthy with all you have gained on the way, not expecting Ithaka to make you rich." The title of this chapter, "While the Light Lasts," acknowledges that darkness will fall as one moves into the final transition "dying." But it also points to the reality that this period has its own work to be done. It both acknowledges that losses move a person into this period of life and resists letting losses *define* this part of the human journey.

The phrase "Work while the light lasts" suggests that the task is being done without artificial light; that something needs urgently to be finished; that the last precious moments are of great value for the desired end result. Think, for example, of farmers using every moment of daylight to finish the harvest. The image of "harvest as day draws to a close," used with care and discretion, may help illumine some otherwise hard-to-see aspects of this time of life. Henri Nouwen (1985, p. 46) asks those entering this period to "trust that the time ahead . . . will be the most important time of your life, not just for you, but for all of us whom you love and who love you."

> After a long struggle during which her daughter moved her into a comfortable assisted-living facility, Honora let go of her resistance to leaving her own home. "I'm so blessed to be here," she said. "There are nice people here, and I'm better off than most." Her room is bright and clean; a few favorite photos decorate the walls; her mother's afghan is on the foot of her bed. Honora is eager to tell you what a gifted life she has had, and how she has no regrets. Her life is different now, but Honora is the same person she always was, and visitors leave her, as visitors always have, with a smile of respect and affection.

Honora would agree with Cavafy, "If you find her poor," that is, if the end of your life brings you to a place that bears little resemblance

---

*KEELEY, EDMUND; *C.P. CAVAFY.* © 1975 by Edmund Keeley and Philip Sherrard. Reprinted by permission of Princeton University Press.

to the journey, do not be surprised. "Ithaka won't have fooled you." In fact, given her health issues, Honora would tell you she is most fortunate to have come to this "Ithaka," as much as she would rather be in her own home. In some sense, it is what she "was destined for," and Honora is realistic enough to know there is no going back, and without the help she has now, her life would be misery for her and for her daughter.

While the broad heterogeneity of the older adult population is narrowed in this period by common elements of dependency and care, conversely the notion of place seems to broaden dramatically. Until recently, place usually referred to the home of a relative, one's own home, or a nursing home. Determination of place was likely linked to socioeconomic or cultural factors. With the increasing size of the older adult population, options regarding place are burgeoning. Many assisted-living facilities offer programs and care tailored to the interests and needs of residents. Some are designed to serve older members of particular minority or ethnic groups, in effect countering decades of tradition in which the care of members of those groups was limited to immediate or extended family. Nor is aging at home what it once was, at least in metropolitan or urban areas: agencies abound that provide the assistance and care needed to make it possible for a person to be comfortably and safely homebound. In fact, communities are being developed where persons living in their own residences can depend on services that address the specific needs of persons in that community, ranging from food preparation to health care, home maintenance, and general errands. Many nursing homes are also providing tailored care, differentiating persons with dementia from those needing physical rehabilitation or postsurgical recovery. A newer trend in nursing home care is to place persons speaking a particular language in proximity to one another. This diversity of options and opportunities explodes many of the traditional (and usually negative) stereotypes of place as the setting for care.

THE ENVIRONMENT OF CARE

Tasks relevant to this period occur and must be understood within the context of an environment of caregiving and some level of dependence on others. This differs in substantial ways from a definition of this period by loss alone. Although dependence on others—whether family members, friends, or professional caregivers—and an environment of caregiving come about by reason of loss, they are at heart relational realities that need to be understood as such.

Giving and receiving care are complex realities, and there is a great difference between one environment of caregiving and another. Some will be optimal, providing "development-enhancing and age-friendly environmental conditions" (Baltes & Baltes, 1990, p. 8); some will be little more than dreadful warehouses for the frail and demented. Most will fall somewhere in between, in large part because our social structures do not provide the resources adequate to respond to the needs of this segment of the population. As Baltes and Baltes (1990) go on to say, "a shift in the balance between gains and losses could be avoided or minimized only if societies were structured in a way that their age-related allocations of resources would fully compensate for the aging loss in 'biological' reserve capacity" (p. 17). The present analysis of the final stable period of life takes social realities into account.

Although this is a stable period, it has a beginning, a middle (potentially long, and with its own shifts and changes), and an end. One enters in frailty and dependency, one ends in dying. Between, there may be months or years—indeed many years—of life that can have their own goals and commitments, their own struggles and joys, their own friendships, freedoms and meaning, their own hardships and pain. "While the Light Lasts" is, after all, a time of life, not death.

The Individual's Experience

People who enter this last stable period of life, "While the Light Lasts," have passed from a normal aging process, which is not characterized by biological or mental pathology, to an aging process dominated (not defined) by losses of physical, mental, or social resources, or to an aging process that is determined by some pathology, such as Alzheimer's disease. There are different sorts of losses, and one's specific losses may profoundly shape an individual's life and differentiate it from others. For example, if the losses are cognitive (as in Alzheimer's disease), the impact of these losses is devastating in ways that physical losses (e.g., mobility, or the ability to transfer oneself from bed to chair) will likely not be. Losses may also be social: a caregiving spouse may die or become incapacitated or a caregiving daughter and her family may have to move to another city because of a job transfer. Such losses can bring about dramatic changes in the way in which dependence on others and the environment of caregiving are shaped and play out.

Although it is possible to generalize about loss, losses specific to each individual can yield very different experiences and outcomes in this final stable period of life. What shape this takes varies greatly from person to person, depending on gender, genetic makeup, environment, financial and social resources, choices that have shaped the individual life course, overall attitude toward life, and what might be described colloquially as "luck of the draw" in using whatever is available to cushion losses. Obviously, the nature of the dependency and the pattern of care will vary dramatically from person to person in intensity, setting, and personnel.

A dominant factor that shapes the particularity of the experience is gender. Women tend to live longer than men, on average by seven years. This means that most women will experience widowhood and, although women tend to replace friendships that are lost in the later years more than do men, they will face rigorous challenges. Economic realities also explain much about the way women experience this time of life differently from men. Women who are now old spent less time in the workplace and were paid less than their male counterparts, leading to dramatically different financial outcomes.

Views of proper care of the elderly may be born by the traditions of individual families or by the larger ethnic heritage in which the family is located. Sociologists have observed that many of these traditions are supported by limited financial resources. In some traditions, the family is obliged to provide the needed care. An African-American friend said, "We would be stigmatized if our mother went to a nursing home." In others, the older person insists upon care delivered by professionals apart from the family. Although it is dangerous to generalize about the care patterns of particular ethnic groups, the notion that "this is how we do it" still dominates in many instances, whether that points to care in a person's home, care in the home of a relative, or care delivered by professionals in a facility designed for that purpose.

Another source of difference is the context in which care is offered: the microcontext, such as home, assisted-living community, or extended-care facility, or the macrocontext, whether one lives in a rural or urban area, in one part of the country or another. Choices of care are limited to opportunities accessible to an individual in a particular place, varying the care experience for each individual by place.

Another important contributor to difference is the background of the individual, both genetic and experiential. Every individual brings a different set of genes to the older adult years. As a result, different individuals will age differently from a physiological perspective. Genetic makeup will frame the physical response to onset of disease as well as the aging process itself. In addition, response to disease is also conditioned by a lifetime of behaviors through which older persons have cared for or abused their bodies. Neither "good genes" nor "staying in shape" assures longevity or freedom from disease, but both are important contributors to the heterogeneity of the experience of the Final Period.

The availability of resources plays a highly significant role in the degree of ease or lack thereof through which the transition to the Final Period is negotiated. These resources may be physical, cognitive, financial, social, or spiritual, and they are distributed differently to each individual. In fact, each person might be placed at a point on a continuum for each of these resources: some will be strong physically, and others very frail. Some will be mentally alert, their memories and cognitive capabilities intact and functioning well, and others will have deteriorating memories and declining reasoning ability. Some will have pension income and the savings of one or more generations, and others will have only their Social Security benefits—or less. Some will have a network of friends and family, relationships high in both quality and quantity, and others will be virtually alone. In making sense of it all, some will be positive in perspective, affirmative in beholding both their own life experience and the future, and others will see so little purpose and meaning that their lives now seem to be little more than a waste.

The Cultural Context

This period suffers in particular ways from negative age stereotyping, heated up by fearful anticipations, unpleasant experiences, and a lack of enough contact with those living in this period to have an adequate basis for judgment. All this makes it hard to see the subtleties and realities of this period of life.

Negative age stereotyping begins with the not-too-subtle premise that the best way to be old is to stay young. The four As of successful aging are active, autonomous, able, alert. Such perceptions ignore the likelihood that over time all will suffer physical losses, probably as the result of disease or disability, and that lifestyles will reflect these losses.

At a deeper level, there is an active disesteem of the old. A leading medical researcher claims, "Aging is nature's way of preparing us for death. That's why we hate old people" (cited in Merkin, 2004, p. 96). Groups of cultural metaphors function to marginalize older adults, particularly those in this period of life. These metaphors focus on aging as physical decline, aging as aesthetic distance from youth, and aging as failure in productivity. It is hard to counter their power (Simmons, 1990). The frail old "sin," egregiously in all three categories, even before the frail old are known as individuals and can be judged on their own humanness. Avis Clendenen (2002) writes of her mother:

> That's what they told me today:
> "In short, she's circling the drain."
> Dwindling
> before my eyes . . .
> I look at her now
> so fragile.
> Hanging on
> but not really.
> "She's circling the drain."
> So succinctly stated;
> but they don't know her
> her life beyond those four words. (p. 110)

Some older persons even marginalize themselves: one person in describing her life in a care facility said she was satisfied with everything, the food, the staff, but that it didn't matter, because her life was over (Gubrium, 1993, p. 58).

A great portion of the adult population sees this period of life through their own fears. No one wants to "end up in a nursing home." No one includes a nursing home in a postretirement agenda. After an adulthood of independence and relative autonomy, the prospect of having to depend on another, even for transportation, let alone for intimate functions such as personal bathing and diaper changing, raises deep fears. What would it be to require assistance? Does it not call into question a person's basic worth, as if every act of care were a reminder of the inability to contribute? A body that refuses to function independently may engender a kind of self-abhorrence that concludes that not only the body but also the whole self is useless and unlovable. This translates into a severe loss of self-esteem, infecting both the present and future.

Disesteem has been fueled in part by some pretty ugly views of nursing-home life. Anna Mae Halgrin Seaver (1994) describes some of her less-than-pleasant experiences as a resident.

> A typical day. Awakened by the woman in the next bed wheezing—a former chain smoker with asthma. Call an aide to wash me and place me in my wheelchair to wait for breakfast. . . . What is today? One day blends into the next until day and date mean nothing. . . . I don't much like some of the physical things that happen to us. I don't care much for a diaper. I seem to have lost the control acquired so diligently as a child. The difference is that I am aware and embarrassed but I can't do anything about it. (p. 11)

Add loss of contact to loss of control and one paints a grim picture. Some environments of care make social contact with persons beyond that environment difficult. One resident of an extended-care facility noted that she had to initiate contact with family members in order to talk with them. Protective barriers that accompany care provided in institutional settings combined with an individual's limited capability may impede the continuation of relationships with persons in the broader community. For various reasons, persons may receive care in facilities distant from their former residence, making them strangers in a strange place, with no friends to visit, a virtual nobody without an identity. Tracy Kidder (1993) observed, "There were no biographies hanging on residents' doors. It was all too apparent that this was a place where biographies ended" (p. 205).

Add also the legitimate uncertainty by which this period is framed. Is the present state of affairs temporary or permanent? Are hopes of recovery of function or mobility realistic or futile? Should I keep my apartment, even though I am currently in an extended-care facility? Will the medical professionals perform one more miracle? Is there a going back? How long will I be a burden? This sense of uncertainty, while it goes with all of the stages of aging, is exacerbated in the Final Period by the person's essential lack of control and dependency on others.

Not all the experiences of the life and circumstances of people in the frailest time of life are negative: a great many persons attest to the quality of care they receive and to the relief that others are engaged in meeting their needs.

Nevertheless, the negative experiences color and dominate perceptions, perhaps because the end of life is often painful. At the end ("the final incapacitating illness") there is likely to be a period of darkness. This may be caused in substantial measure because today so many deaths—typically from cancer, congestive heart failure, or chronic obstructive pulmonary disease—are long and slow, and many people endure substantial pain during their last days. According to a study published in the *Journal of the American Medical Association,* 40 percent of nursing-home patients with chronic or acute pain are not receiving treatment to relieve it, a further indication that the pain management needs of elderly patients are frequently overlooked (cited in Stedman, 2002, p. 154).

The pictures from those who have had extended contact with people in this period of life are likely to be much more nuanced than are those from a distance. Most citizens simply do not have enough experience with people in this period to have an adequate picture of this world. The same could be said, perhaps, of other groups—for example, the world of third graders—but the key difference in our lack of knowledge relates to where most adults are headed. It is not to the third grade!

Dark Shadows of Care

Other issues related to the need for care and derived from the inability to function independently that can cast a shadow over this period include neglect and elder abuse. Add grieving and the loss of self-esteem to the essential loss of independence and one has the recipe for depression. Estimates of the rate of depression among residents of nursing homes range from 1 in 10 to 1 in 2. According to the National Institutes of Health, up to 15 percent of older adults have clinically significant depressive symptoms, and up to 25 percent of nursing-home residents suffer from the disorder (National Institutes of Health, 1991). Similar rates have been projected for homebound elderly. Not unrelated is the prevalence of depression in family members dealing with the strain and responsibility of caregiving. According to testimony before the Senate Special Committee on Aging, "depression occurs in more than 60 percent of wives, 40 percent of husbands, 40 percent of daughters and daughter-in-laws, 25 percent of sons, and 25 percent of other relatives caring for relatives with dementia at home" (Cohen, 2003). In some instances, the stress of caregiving results in incidents of elder abuse and neglect among older adults, especially women who are depressed, confused, or frail and who live in their own homes. Perpetrators of abuse or neglect tend to be family members, particularly adult children or spouses (Administration on Aging, 1997).

THE CHALLENGE FOR THE PROFESSIONAL

As a person enters this Final Period of life, the diversity of opportunities experienced in earlier periods is greatly reduced as an individual is introduced into a continuum of care, and life seems to have a narrower range of possibilities. This focuses the role of professionals, caregivers, family members, and other support personnel. With increasing dependency, their supportive roles are magnified in importance when the older adult has little agency apart from those engaged in supportive, professional, or caregiving roles. As an older adult's circle of relationships, both formal and informal, becomes smaller, the role of those who remain, whether professionals, friends, or family members, grows larger.

Although many of the roles that professionals and other support persons have assumed in prior periods—expertise, advocacy, and loving care—remain, there are several challenges that are highlighted by this period.

One is to view the person receiving care as a unique individual, rather than as a member of a class of disabled persons. For example, some individuals are mentally alert but physically impaired, while others are physically able but mentally compromised by illness or medication. Some have very intact memories, while others have lost their short-term memories entirely. Each is a participant in a family tradition as well as a cultural tradition. Strengths and capabilities should be identified and utilized within the context of a person's traditions. Preconceived notions of persons' mental, physical, and emotional health impede both the caregiving process and professional relationships. To engage in a relationship with a person in this period capitalizing on whatever abilities are available is to do that person a great service.

Examples of this can be seen in the best facilities where people care for those with late-stage Alzheimer's disease. Caregiving professionals in these units characteristically treat those for whom they care with gracious attention, humor, and an awareness of the spiritual struggles and challenges of this disease. It is against this level of excellence that all professional caregiving has to be measured.

It is estimated that of the approximately 1 million Americans living currently in assisted-living residences, at least half of them have some form of dementia (Basler, 2006, p. 16). Against this background, many extended-care facilities explore new ways to customize care for the individual, encourage independence, engage in interesting and productive activities, and maintain a comfortable, homelike, and noninstitutional atmosphere. Professionals as well as family members and other caregivers are obliged to keep current with the latest in extended-care opportunities as options increase in both variety and effectiveness.

Another challenge is to provide advocacy for adequate levels of care. Sometimes this takes the form of recommending sufficient pain management and palliative care to provide comfort. Fully half of all hospitalized patients have moderate to severe pain in their last days of life, and patients in nursing homes are very likely to experience untreated pain. Furthermore, pain experienced by blacks and Hispanics was more likely to be undertreated than pain experienced by whites (Robert Wood Johnson Foundation, 2006).

Many older persons, particularly members of minority groups or persons without health insurance or financial resources, are the products of lifetimes in which professional health care services have been underutilized. This may be the result of unequal access, lack of information, lack of affordability, or cultural factors that emphasize alternative healing strategies. In any case, advocacy may take the form of encouraging appropriate use of health care services designed for persons in need of end-of-life care.

In other instances advocacy may take the form of distinguishing diseases (which are treatable) from the aging process (which is not a disease). To refrain from providing treatment simply because a person is "old and will likely die before long anyway" is to make aging a disease from which there is no recovery and for which there is no treatment. According to an article titled "The Quality of Medical Care Provided to Vulnerable Community-Dwelling Older Patients" published in *Annals of Internal Medicine,* for specific geriatric conditions, physicians provided the clinically recommended treatments in only a limited percentage of instances in the following sample of conditions: malnutrition, 47 percent of the time; pressure ulcers, 41 percent; dementia, 35 percent; fall and mobility disorders, 34 percent; urinary incontinence, 29 percent (Wenger et al., 2003).

Concerns expressed by persons in this period, according to a 2002 study that appeared in the *New England Journal of Medicine,* most frequently mentioned diminished autonomy, declining capacity to take part in enjoyable activities, and the fear of losing control over bodily functions. Howard Moody (2003) comments that these concerns "point to suffering, rather than pain, as the key to end-of-life care" and underscore the loss of meaning and dignity that often accompany contemporary health care (p. 2). This may be particularly true where a hospital ethos of cure overwhelms a commonsense awareness of the need simply for care.

One often overlooked challenge is the need to facilitate communication with the person receiving care and with family members and others. Communication includes information about care and treatment as well as sharing issues, concerns, and personal messages. The role of communication has as its purpose not only to dispel misinformation, but also to encourage all parties to be open in addressing end-of-life topics that many would be inclined to avoid.

An important aspect of such openness in communication is basic honesty about what is happening to the older person's body. When the description of a person's physical well-being is shrouded in euphemisms and other language that camouflages the truth, significant changes will often surprise both the patient and family alike and find them unprepared for new eventualities.

Depending on the extent of planning that has occurred in earlier periods, the task of addressing end-of-life issues may be modest, or it may be great. A change in circumstances since earlier plans were laid may also impact this task: for example, the cost of care may have depleted the financial resources upon which earlier plans were based. Relationships with family members and others may have changed during the recent years. Issues ranging from levels of care (usually described in advance directives) to celebration of one's life at death (usually contained in plans or wishes for one's funeral or memorial service) will inevitably confront. The time is approaching when these end-of-life decisions will be required, whether or not they have been carefully made.

Changes in understanding plus the introduction of specific circumstances since advance directives were formulated may involve professionals in interpreting those directives in the present situation. Many decisions must be made at the intersection of advance directives, the policy of the institution or provider, and the will of members of the family, and involve difficult decisions such as whether to request or refuse a "do not resuscitate" order or artificial nutrition and hydration. Professionals may find themselves in circumstances where the family may not agree with a person's advance directives, or where the family and patient are at odds with the health care provider, and may need to assist the family or other caregivers to understand and address such issues.

BEING OKAY AMID DEPENDENCY AND FRAILTY

How can it be that there are people who are quite sick, frail, and dependent who are nevertheless happy, committed, generous, satisfied—who are, in a word, okay?

A leading theory of life span development proposes that individuals manage their lives successfully through three processes:

1. Selecting or setting goals that are important to them ("I know exactly what I want and what I don't want.")

2. Optimizing choices to get to these goals ("I make every effort to achieve a given goal.")
3. Compensating when they cannot manage their activities as they used to ("When things aren't going so well I accept help from others.") (Freund & Baltes, 2002, pp. 661-662)

These findings came from a larger study on adult personality involving heterogeneous (in occupation and education) samples from the greater Berlin, Germany, area. The authors note that although the use of these life management strategies increased over adulthood, they declined somewhat in old age because of physical and biological constraints, given the effort and resource-dependent nature of this life management tool.

It makes sense intuitively that, in general, people of all ages who scored well in each of these three areas of life management were happier and more satisfied with their lives than those who scored less well. But this is an important and empirically validated finding.

Lifelong, people engage in the process of selecting goals from the many opportunities that are presented. Life requires choices so that people can focus their energy and actually accomplish something. In late frail age, the number of options available may be fewer, and the biological and physical constraints might make this process more difficult to achieve and less likely to be helpful. But—and this surprised the authors of this study—the indication is that as people get older they get better at selecting elective life goals that are satisfying to them. This ability to refine one's life goals is one key to life satisfaction, whether the setting of goals is simply from one's own choice or in response to a loss (Freund & Baltes, 2002).

A second mechanism of okayness in dependence and frailty is referred to as a shift from tenacious goal pursuit to flexible goal adjustment, with a focus more on compensating. Put simply, older people reality-test their likelihood of achieving their goals. When they know the goals are out of reach, they choose new goals—and accept a little help along the way. People do adjust to irreversible changes and losses. Sometimes, people can change the situation so that it is acceptable. They learn new ways of managing or accommodating. They change routines, they leave more time for tasks, they find appropriate assistive devices, they let someone help them with bathing or dressing, and so on (an assimilative mode of coping). The interplay between accommodation and assimilation shifts with age. One study concluded that in later adulthood "Tenacious Goal Pursuit decreases with age, and Flexible Goal Adjustment shows a clear increase" (Brandstädter & Baltes-Götz, 1990, p. 220).

At other times, people find that it is simply too difficult to control the situation. In order to be okay emotionally, they learn to reassess their options and adjust their wants and aspirations to more manageable levels (an accommodative mode of coping). Gilbert Brim (1988) describes his father's activity during this time:

> In dealing with the gaps between his aspirations and achievements, he altered his methods, such as adding help, both personal and mechanical; he lowered his level of aspiration, being willing to settle for less; and he shifted goals as he grew older. (p. 51)

Satisfaction from Adjustments

What may be hard to imagine from a younger age is that this state of affairs is happy or emotionally satisfying. Brandstädter and Baltes-Götz (1990) (citing an earlier work by Mayring) concluded,

> The compensatory shift from assimilative toward more accommodative styles of coping may help to stabilize the subjective balance of developmental gains and losses over the life span; thus, it may account for the fact that age-comparative studies to date have not been able to document a general deterioration of personal satisfaction and well-being in later life. (pp. 220-221)

It is a point worth careful attention.

Missouri author Adele Starbird writes about a visit with her mother in a nursing home, in which her mother began:

> "Well, things are going well for me . . . I am on an entirely new track. I'm just trying to be pleasant all the time."
>
> "Is it a great effort?"
>
> "Did you ever try it?"
>
> "No, I am going to wait until I'm your age before trying anything so drastic."

"It's the only thing that's left now that I can do for anybody. I can't read or write, but I can at least be pleasant and not add to the troubles of others. You know I think that every human being is already carrying about as much as he can bear, and I don't want to make it harder." (cited in Carnahan, 2002, p. 1)

The author concludes: "Pleasant. She was more than pleasant—she was gallant" (Carnahan, 2002, p. 1).

Objective Realities and Subjective Responses

Baltes and Baltes (1990) describe two aspects of aging that in real lives are inextricably intertwined: the *objective* aspects of medical, psychological, and social functioning and the *subjective* aspects of quality of life and meaning. People may cope with a great deal of negative objective aspects of aging and still have a quality of life that allows them to describe themselves as happy and productive. For example, one woman writes, "For the most [part], being positive is three-fourths of the battle—accepting the unacceptable and acknowledging and working from my strengths amid my vivid disabilities and weaknesses." When asked to name the best thing about being 94, a wheelchair-bound woman in a hospital answered without hesitation, "No peer pressure" (Metropolitan Diary, 1998, p. A18).

One investigator (Field, 1997) asked people aged 73 to 93, "Looking back, what period of life brought you the most satisfaction?" In spite of the bias of her question ("looking *back*"), to her surprise, more than a third said, "Right now."

Describing nursing-home residents, Elizabeth MacKinlay (2001) notes,

> Somehow, the reality did not seem as bad as the perception. These people were already frail, living with more than one chronic illness and vulnerable in a number of ways. Of this group, 45 percent expressed some fears, a much lower proportion than those living independently (100 percent). In fact, 55 percent said they had no fears at all. Yet the people in this study were much more frail and required assistance in several of the activities of daily living. They were in fact experiencing the

very things that those living in the community held as future fears. (p. 158)

How one views one's life and well-being generally emerges in contrasting one's ideal with one's actual self-conception. Heidrich (1994) found the disparity between actual and ideal to be more predictive of depression among elderly women than their physical health status. This theoretical construct provides two options for accommodation in order to enhance well-being: a person may adjust one's ideal view in order to be more congruent with the actual, or one may seek to improve one's actual situation in order to be more congruous with the ideal. Older persons have a lifetime of experience adjusting by learning to live with situations they cannot change.

Baltes and Baltes (1990) conclude:

> Because of a negative aging stereotype, one might easily expect that older persons would hold less positive views of themselves and their efficacy to control their own lives. Contradictory to this expectation, however, old people on the average do not differ from young people in reports of their subjective life satisfaction or on self-related measures such as personal control or self-efficacy. (p. 18)

While it is true that, with aging, the balance between gains and losses becomes less positive, it is also true that the self remains amazingly resilient in old age.

THE BLESSING OF CARE

Henri Nouwen (1985) claims that the last days of one's life are the most important ones (p. 46). Despite the fact of loss, most persons still believe their lives to be worthwhile and purposeful. This perspective stands in sharp contrast to the common view that these are "throwaway" days, and those requiring care are expendable people.

Care is a word whose meaning carries more than one inference. As part of the everyday vocabulary, care is synonymous with great interest or deep concern. In suggesting affection or love, it also connotes some level of reciprocity or mutuality: "We care for each other." When one's body suffers debilitation, or one is unable to contribute to the daily activities of a household, or when one is no longer physically able to care for another, it may be difficult to believe that another cares. Signs and demonstrations of love and friendship that bridge isolation and provide support and reassurance remind one of the sustaining value of life and love, even under difficult circumstances.

The other meaning of care, as in "to take care of," has become synonymous in many minds with personal inadequacy and indignity. Care in this context is a constant reminder of a person's insufficiency. It undermines self-confidence, as it demonstrates the very opposite of mutuality. The one engaged in the intimate business of caring—known officially as a caregiver—may be a spouse or a family member. The spouse or sibling as caregiver may be about the same age as the one being cared for and may also suffer problems with physical and mental health. Or it may be a stranger who may be like the one receiving care, or who may be different in terms of age, gender, race, class, or upbringing and expectations.

Responding to care, developing a life within the context of care, and relating to a caregiver who may be a relative or a stranger challenges one to enlarge the view of those who are important in life. Instead of simply representing insufficiency and indignity, caregiving also provides the tools for support and comfort and the means to live. It is easy to wish that life had not come to this. Indeed, a great many are genuinely surprised that it has. But to look the present in the face, and reject those cultural norms that idolize sufficiency, is to ascribe to caregiving the virtue that it allows older persons to continue the journey.

ENGAGING AND DISENGAGING

The need for care and the presence of regular caregivers do not erase the need for conversation, companionship, and support. Is there a life not enriched by being connected to others who share mutual regard and compassion? It is not surprising that studies suggest that older persons prefer friends of many years to newer friends. However, one of the elements of loss experienced in the latter years is the loss of friends through death, relocation, or confinement. The litany for many in this stage is, "All my friends are gone." The fact is further complicated by the increasing difficulty one has in making friends when one is in a state of dependency or disability. In fact, some believe that friendship is based only on sharing expectations for the future, and when one becomes old, there is no clear future, few expectations, and, therefore, nothing upon which to base a friendship (Kaufman, 1986, p. 110). Although it may never be too late to make new friends, or to make younger friends, or to reconstruct one's support network, it becomes increasingly more challenging to do so as the effects of multiple transitions accumulate.

Two other factors add to the difficulty in maintaining relationships at this time. For nearly half a century scholars have debated whether aging is synonymous with a mutual withdrawal or disengagement, a theory describing decreased interaction between a person and others in the social systems to which the person belongs (Cumming & Henry, 1961). Given the circumstances of age and dependence, some inclination toward disengagement and decreased interaction may be expected, posing an obstacle to developing and continuing relationships. Nursing homes have been described as settings "where potential social partners are abundant but interaction rates are strikingly low," explained in part by withdrawal as a response to overcrowded and unpredictable social environments (Carstensen, 2001, p. 270). Bassuk, Glass, and Berkman (1999) have demonstrated a relationship between social disengagement and cognitive decline in community-dwelling elders. They found that persons with no social ties, when compared with others who had five or six social ties, were at increased risk for cognitive decline. Others (Haan, 1999) have suggested that social contact, rather than declining, simply changes and becomes more fluid as organizations become involved with providing care, as the role of the family changes, or as the measure of significance of social contact is transmuted from frequency of contact to level of instrumental and emotional support it provides.

Other older persons, when asked to reflect on their own disengagement, see it as a broader function and list areas where they have disengaged as well as areas where they have engaged or reengaged. A friend described how, after the last major disagreement at church, he disengaged from the congregation, but how he has begun the practice of telephoning some individuals with whom he used to have more frequent interaction. Care must always be used in interpreting such findings, lest presumptions of cause and effect confound descriptions of behaviors that occur simultaneously. One might more safely conclude that the Final Period as a whole involves any number of changes that occur in the area of a person's relationships and social contacts, as well as in the broader areas of physical, mental, emotional, and social health, and the Later Transition proceeds with different rates and patterns among different individuals.

A second factor is drawn from "exchange theory" that assumes that relationships are based on the premise of mutuality: both participants contribute and both profit, and the benefits of such a relationship outweigh the costs to both participants. However, when one participant is dependent or confined, it may be hard to discern what that one may contribute to a friendship beyond a smile or greeting. Furthermore, in the case of intergenerational relationships, members of the older generation may be more invested in the younger generation than vice versa (Walker et al., 2001, p. 18), making it more difficult for the older participant to maintain the relationship. The perception that being marginalized is inevitable may lead persons in this period to be less assertive in maintaining relationships. One elderly nursing-home resident noted that in those instances where she feels that she is the one who always makes the phone calls, she is inclined to stop calling. She said, "If they really wanted to talk with me, they would call once in a while, too."

Difficulties notwithstanding, persons in this final stable period of life are able to maintain relationships with family and friends, are able to initiate new relationships—often with others who are also recipients of care, or with those who are caregivers. In recent years, some nursing homes and assisted-living facilities have installed personal computers and provided instruction in their use to enable residents to maintain contact with family and friends.

Of course, not all relationships depend on mail, whether paper-based or electronic. Recently, a local newspaper portrayed a 96-year-old gentleman with his 95-year-old bride being wed by the mayor of the town where they were residents of an extended-care home. The caption described them as the world's oldest newlyweds. Friendships blossom in all circumstances and environments so long as there is a positive attitude about expanding the circle to include others.

IS AUTONOMY A CONTRADICTION?

To speak of autonomy or control within a care environment seems a contradiction. The introduction of care may appear to preclude any notions of independence. How can one be in control, deciding what to do, where to live, and with whom to associate, when in order to live one is in the care of persons who make or greatly influence many of those decisions. This issue is most acute in the case of an involuntary confinement in a nursing-home situation or complete dependence on a caregiver at home; less acute when a nursing home has, however reluctantly, been the individual's choice; even less acute in an assisted-living facility where there is greater freedom; and still less acute when the level of dependency is modest (but real).

After a half century of self-directing adulthood, it is difficult to admit that one has reached a point where complete self-reliance is no longer a possibility. The deleterious impact on the ego may be more than an individual can manage. For many, a sense of being a person is clearly bound up with a sense of control. Years of professional responsibility as well as personal leadership have reinforced the notion of being in charge, if not of others, at least of oneself. In many instances, older persons describe their dependency as a temporary state, expecting to regain health and, with it, independence. Whether this represents genuine hope or is simply a way to avoid dealing with the damage dependency has done to the ego is impossible to ascertain. For with the introduction of care, not only is this self-image challenged, but also the fundamental integrity of the person as well. Reluctance to receiving care may be a veiled, or not so veiled, resistance to being overly dependent on others and the loss of personal power involved.

Opportunities for decision making and self-advocacy are often neglected in a care culture where the norm is passivity. A nursing-home resident said that he didn't need to read because others read for him. "In fact," he said, "I don't even have to think about things, because they do that for me too." "Not to decide" can become the default option, although competent caregivers are aware that the mental and physical health of those in their care is enhanced by their participation in decision-making processes about matters great and small. Depending on residents for decision making is one of the marks of progressive care in assisted-living and extended-care communities. Many studies have drawn connections between the degree of control people have felt over their lives and their longevity.

Giving Up Control

With control goes a measure of health of body and spirit. But there can also be a sense of well-being that goes with giving up control. Giving it up, rather than having it taken away. Giving up control is not synonymous with giving up on life, although it may be for a few. Giving up control means getting out of the way of one's progress. A life review may bring to mind those times when in the wake of stepping aside, real progress followed. It means setting some portion of one's ego on the shelf, not fretting the small stuff. For many, giving up control has spiritual dimensions, recognizing the illusory nature of control, the underlying foundations of faith, and that at any age or circumstance, there is much that cannot be controlled or managed. To be preoccupied with ego is to waste valuable energy that could more productively be devoted to the business of living.

The irony of control is that what is dominated also enslaves. The paradox of control is that in giving it up, real freedom results. Freedom comes from simplifying, from concentrating on the essentials; it comes from giving up lifelong conventions and long lists of oughts. It results in relaxation, exemption from old chores, time to enjoy, and a look toward the present instead of the past. Or as John Kenneth Galbraith said, "I've made one concession to great age: to know there are some things I can ignore" (Terkel, 1995, p. 329).

WHAT'S THE POINT?

Most questions at this stage of aging, particularly if time spent in it is very long, may be reduced to this one: What's the point? Is there purpose to these days? Is it possible for a person suffering serious disability or frailty to find meaning, achieve goals, and continue to follow a productive and fruitful path? What does fruitfulness and productivity mean for a person who may be dependent on others for care?

More than one person receiving extensive care has voiced the notion that he or she has lived too long already. One woman said to those sitting on the park bench with her:

> I worry about my friends. They're all suffering. Tillie can't see so good and has a double hernia. Helen needs a new hip and lives on Nuprin and Advil. What's the point? I ask you again, what's the point? (Norman, 1996, p. 38)

By way of affirmation, Carl Jung (1933) argues that

> a human being would certainly not grow to be seventy or eighty years old if this longevity had no meaning for the species to which he belongs. The afternoon of human life must also have a significance of its own and cannot be merely a pitiful appendage to life's morning. (p. 109)

Henri Nouwen (1985) writes:

> To care for . . . the many who can no longer expect to return to their work, who can no longer be of service to their families and friends, is to search together for new meaning, a meaning no longer drawn from activities to get things done. Somehow, meaning must grow out of the "passivities" of waiting. . . . Believing that our lives come to fulfillment in dependence requires a tremendous leap of faith. (pp. 90, 93)

Quest for Meaning

Whether based on faith in a divine being or faith in oneself, the quest for meaning takes on two dimensions, one internal, the other external. And the quest takes on some urgency, as the time clock of mortality and the opportunities it represents tick away. The internal quest for meaning seeks to make sense of the present, affirm the past, and pull the two together into a cohesive whole, confident that the journey has not ended. Erik Erikson (1950) called this ego integrity. By whatever name, it is based on a fundamental sense of self-worth and dignity and involves the giant task of connecting past with present, the reasonable with the absurd, and gathering, in the words of Malcolm Boyd (2001), "fragments of our lives into a pattern of wholeness" (p. 56).

The process takes place through reflection, through conversation, and through the construction, formal or informal, of one's own life review. Webster and Young (1988) point out that the life review process may represent an "adaptive restructuring of the personality in the face of stress or impending death" (p. 318). Cohler (1993), citing Erikson and Butler, describes the function of memory in life review as often performing the function previously performed by being with others. He also highlights the importance of a remembered past for the maintenance of morale in the present. Life review balances the positive with the not-so-positive, and provides an opportunity for finding answers and discovering peace. It may be written or spoken, and for some it is taken through the pathways of the mind.

But the function of meaning-making, in addition to coming to terms with the past, is to discover anew a reason for living in the present. By looking at oneself, as if for the first time, a person is able to discover a purpose, whether through the development of goals expressly for this time of life or for adaptation of goals long held. New goals may be as simple and straightforward as maintaining the brain as a well-functioning organ through continued learning via a regimen of reading, games, and discussion, or of talking with the grandchildren when they come from school, or as complex as completing one's autobiography, or writing the family history or creating a work of art. The time presents still another opportunity to reinvent oneself in various ways.

It also provides the opportunity for winding up the unfinished business of a lifetime: getting one's affairs in order, renewing and repairing relationships, planning one's legacy, discussing how one's life is to be celebrated, distributing special possessions, and telling the story that goes with each of them. It is a time to affirm past achievements, put aside the guilt from past failures, and assess what one passes on when one passes on. George Vaillant (2002) says that "positive aging means to love, to work, to learn something we did not know yesterday, and to enjoy the remaining precious moments with loved ones" (p. 16). Robert Frost (1930) captures the imperative of these days in lines from "Stopping by Woods on a Snowy Evening":

> But I have promises to keep,
> And miles to go before I sleep . . .

Many have argued that these are important days, the time when the modulation toward life's final tonic chord begins.

But meaning is about more than choosing appropriate activities. It is about drawing conclusions about the past, the present, and the future, and endeavoring to live those conclusions. For some, the present situation, often involving suffering of body, mind, or spirit displays life as a waste at its worst. For others, suffering is an opportunity for grace, a potential blessing with spiritual dimensions. It is a religious experience that is not only designed to improve persons, but is also a means by which lives are sanctified and made holy.

Professionals, caregivers, family members, and others fail the individual in this Final Period when they intentionally avoid or under the press of time neglect the spiritual dimension of aging. Some have affirmed that it is impossible to help an older person without understanding that a person's spiritual journey provides the context for decision making and care. Engaging a person at this level is less about religion and more about affirming meaning through listening and sustaining a person with empathy. At root, engaging a person spiritually is advocacy at its best, that is, "standing with" the other whether in celebrating life or facing the mystery of death. It is therefore ill-advised for professionals either to assume the meaning attached to the experiences of this Final Period or to impose theirs.

Making a Difference

Nevertheless, the pursuit of purpose need not be directed entirely to the internal. In activities focused on the community and the world, this time represents one of the last chances to make a difference.

> At 94, confined to a wheelchair and quite unable to accomplish many of the basic tasks of daily living, Dan spent time each day visiting the other people in his world. Whatever the other's stage of decline or "disrepair" Dan's smile was the same. His tender and welcoming "How are you today?" was an invitation to speak freely to this good listener. At his death, the sense of loss among staff and residents was so real that a grief counselor was brought in.

Dan demonstrates that the final stable period of life can serve as a powerful motivating tool to make a difference both to oneself and to one's community. Not everyone's abilities or opportunities are the same. Many can do more; many must do less. All can envision a difference they can make in the lives of others, whether through the use of their talents, their resources, or their influence—and can pass on something of worth. Henri Nouwen (1985) cautions against being concerned with immediate accomplishments and influence, and encourages looking long term: "How can I live so that I can continue to be fruitful when I am no longer here among my family and friends? That questions shifts our attention from doing to being" (p. 41).

JOURNEYING ON

The horizon diminishes, the issues and needs become short term and close at hand. Yet in his poem "An Ancient to Ancients," Thomas Hardy speaks of the elderly who "burnt brightlier toward their setting day" (cited in Meyerhoff, 1978, p. xii). But bright or not, the journey continues. The spirit of the time is aptly caught by the words from Leonard Bernstein's *Mass* ("I Go On" text by Stephen Schwartz and Leonard Bernstein):

> When the thunder rumbles,
> Now the Age of Gold is dead
> And the dreams we've clung to dying to stay young
> Have left us parched and old instead,
> When my courage crumbles,
> When I feel confused and frail,
> When my spirit falters on decaying alters
> And my illusions fail,
> I go on right then,
> I go on again.
> I go on to say I will celebrate another day.
> I go on.
> If tomorrow tumbles
> And everything I love is gone,
> I will face regret
> All my days, and yet I will still go on.
> Lauda, Lauda, Laude.

Chapter 8

Dying Well

"Dying" refers to the actual transition from life to death. The end point of the transition is clear physically—a last breath is taken, a human heart stops beating, a person becomes lifeless. Yet these simple physical facts cloak a great mystery—no one reports from beyond death on what kind of experience it was, or what human meaning that final human act had for the person who made that transition. In all the other transitions and stable periods along the way, those who go ahead can say what lies in the future. In "dying" there is only silence at the end, interpreted through the tradition in which one lives. Nonetheless, the transition is long enough and complex enough that there is much to learn about it—except for its denouement.

The name for this chapter, "Dying Well," is inspired by the work of Ira Byock, MD, and his book *Dying Well: The Prospect for Growth at the End of Life* (1997a) that focuses on dying as a continuous process rather than simply the moment of death. Dying well means that pain is controlled, that fear and loneliness are reduced, and that death is approached and engaged as a natural part of human life that, like other parts, can promote growth and understanding. Dying well also assumes that the full experience of dying is not captured by a purely medical perspective. To die well is to reach certain landmarks: asking forgiveness, accepting forgiveness, expressing love, acknowledging self-worth, and saying good-bye. In the final part of the transition, dying well also means letting go, surrendering to the transcendent, to the unknown.

A Journey Called Aging: Challenges and Opportunities in Older Adulthood
© 2007 by The Haworth Press, Taylor & Francis Group. All rights reserved.
doi:10.1300/5915_09 *191*

THE BEGINNING

The beginning point of the transition is not always clear, even physically. Something happens. There is a turn for the worse. Some physical signal—perhaps as clear as a doctor's use of the word *terminal,* perhaps something more subtle and personal—tells this person that this illness is "unto death." One's face is, for a reason that may not be fully understood or articulated, turned toward the setting sun. Bodily systems fail to function at prior levels; perhaps cognition declines. Sometimes the person's contact with the environment and those in it becomes inconsistent.

In some instances and cultures, the older person seems to provide the initiative, making dying an intentional act. Murray Trelease (1975) tells of his work as an Episcopal priest among native populations in Alaska:

> A young member of a family would come to my cabin and ask me to come pray for grandma and bring Communion. And when I arrived the whole family and close friends would be there and we would have a service together. Within hours after that, the person would be dead . . . most often it was the one dying who called everyone together. And I was told on several occasions that the dying person had spent the past few days making plans, telling the story of his life and praying for all the members of the family. (p. 34)

In most instances, however, dying simply happens to a person, or so it is generally perceived. The process ushers in a series of developmental tasks that begins with a sense of completion with worldly affairs and ends with the surrender of all (Byock, 1997b).

A spouse or adult child may make the transition more difficult to accept by refusing to acknowledge the reality that the person entering the transition is trying to claim and understand. Persistent good wishes for getting well and feeling better may appear to withhold permission for continuing the journey unto death. The refusal of families and friends to "let go" is often reinforced by institutions such as hospitals, where the prevailing culture of cure focuses on recovery, and where care to the exclusion of cure is rejected as failure. Death-denying aspects of contemporary Western culture prompt efforts to microman-age death as if it were little more than another task to be accomplished or an option to be selected.

Death is certain; the time of death is uncertain. This distinction clearly differentiates this transition from the others. Death can hap-pen in one's thirties or forties or fifties or on the eighteenth green in the prime of Extended Middle Age. But none of these will be the same as death after all life's other stages have fully run their courses. Death in earlier years carries with it a sense of injustice, of a wrong that could have been averted with appropriate care in living and proper medical attention. In a graveyard in Tidewater, Virginia, a re-cent gravestone with the dates of the woman's brief life is engraved with the words, "I told you I was sick." Death before its time invites outrage and struggle. As Dylan Thomas (1945) writes:

> And you, my father, there on the sad height,
> Curse, bless, me now with your fierce tears, I pray.
> Do not go gentle into that good night.
> Rage, rage against the dying of the light. (p. 207)

Death in late life has its own dynamics:

> By the time people reach their late 80s or 90s, they have experi-enced multiple losses. Most are widowed, and, in addition, they have lost most if not all their siblings and closest friends. Although these losses are important ones, leaving feelings of great sadness, . . . oldest old adults experience such losses as in-evitable at their stage of life. These on-time losses, then, do not have as extensive an impact as we might think when we look at them from the frame of our own developmental understanding. (Walker et al., p. 238)

Thoughts of mortality, or perhaps the simple recognition that one is not immortal, beginning as early as middle age, continue over the years and multiply. From infrequent visitor, these thoughts become a persistent guest. In each of the stages in the framework of older adult development, death becomes more of a concern, until, finally, it be-comes a present reality. Instead of a stage to be programmed neatly into a framework, it has become an intervention or interruption that seems to hover and can occur at any time. The average longevity data for the United States suggest that, on average, death comes in the mid-to-late seventies, earlier for men, later for women, depending on the year of birth. For a great many, death occurs during the Early Transition or the Older Adult Lifestyle period. But since this is the average, death will also occur earlier, during Extended Middle Age for some, and later, during Later Transition and the Final Period, or While the Light Lasts, for others. The location of this chapter on dying at the end of the book does not necessarily mean that a person must or will progress through all of the stages and transitions of older adulthood in order to reach it. Instead, death comes to reach us. A great many persons in every stage of development have accepted the inevitability of their own death: some are prepared, even eager, but others find it an impossible topic to consider.

Whether death is at the end of a life course (a death in due season) or death comes early in life (a death out of season) the core defining reality is the same: dying is a powerful and final part of every human life.

THE MEDICALIZATION OF DYING

Dying is not made easier for being on time, however, if the quality of care is poor or inappropriate. In the fall of 2000, Public Affairs Television aired a series hosted by Bill Moyers, *On Our Own Terms: Moyers on Dying in America.* In a letter introducing the series, Moyers (2000) wrote:

> Modern advances in medicine and profound social changes have prolonged life but also transformed the experience of dying. While 90 percent of Americans say they want to die at home, four out of five of us will die in a hospital or other healthcare facility. Many die in needless pain, and because the dying process takes longer, it exacts a greater toll on individuals, families, caregivers and communities. (p. 2)

The four major influences on death and dying that dominate U.S. culture, even when one is attentive to the very pluralistic reality of society (Kaufman, 1998), are

1. medicine has become the dominant framework for understanding dying and death;

2. technology is allowed to determine end-of-life events;
3. people engaged in care often have competing goals for end-of-life care; and
4. few people are knowledgeable about available technology and are prepared to share in decisions about technology's uses.

Even within a medical system, the ethos of *cure* clashes with and dominates an ethos of *care,* often without regard to the needs of the dying person. There is no compelling alternative to cure in the medical model. "In the historical development of clinical medicine, the primacy of the discourse of curing has marginalized the discourses of comforting and caring" (Pierson, 2000, p. 233). Medicare regulations currently allow terminally ill persons to receive medical treatment and chemotherapy while receiving hospice benefits, further extending the element of cure into the sanctuary of the dying.

It is a mark of contemporary Western culture—whatever progress is being made in open and constructive conversation about dying—that death is medicalized, a term that comes from Ivan Illich's (1976) critique. The medicalization of dying includes a

> loss of the capacity to accept death and suffering as meaningful aspects of life; a sense of being in a state of "total war" against death at all stages of the life cycle; a crippling of personal and family care, and a devaluing of traditional rituals surrounding dying and death. (Clark, 2002, p. 905)

The issue is less about whether medical care is helpful, even necessary, and more about whether its main purpose is to postpone dying. In an earlier chapter, concern was expressed about the uneven quality of health care available to older adults. This chapter argues for care of the highest quality but, as appropriate, palliative care consistent with the needs and wishes of the patient rather than those of caregiver or medical personnel.

Clark (2002) goes further in his analysis:

> Yet just as palliative care has encouraged medicine to be gentler in its acceptance of death, parallel developments in the medical system have redoubled efforts in the opposite direction. One aspect of this is the problem of futile treatments that either have

a low probability of having an effect or produce an effect that is of no benefit to the patient. Further problems derive from the widespread assumption in society that every cause of death can be resisted, postponed, or avoided. (p. 905)

More than 25 years after Illich's critique, a friend wrote,

Dad had a stroke and was 11 weeks in intensive care and then a step-down unit, and then died rather suddenly with none of us with him, although we had been with him through those weeks, as much as they would let us.

In this view, death results from the failure of science and human will to master the environment. If every death is contingent, a matter of chance, there is no reason why any particular injury or disease cannot be overcome by medical science. When death is thus medicalized, it is transformed. Recently, a frail woman who had made careful decisions with her family about her own care at the end of her life experienced a bout of severe shortness of breath. Rather than use the oxygen at hand to alleviate her distress, the family panicked and called 911. After enduring the horrors of 51 days in intensive care, she was released to a comfort-care-only convalescent home. She died three days later. In intensive care, physicians and medical staff had tried to do what they were trained to do: cure disease, prolong life, and restore function. In this model, the implicit assumption is that improved quality of life can be attained only by curing what is wrong, not—as was needed in this case—by providing an environment in which a person can die well, relieved of suffering.

It was only a few decades ago that Elisabeth Kübler-Ross (1969) reported that she could not find dying patients to interview in the hospital in which she worked if she relied on physicians for referral. None of their patients was dying! But her description of the five steps in the process by which persons come to terms with their own immanent death has become one of several frameworks for responding to the news on one's impending death. According to Kübler-Ross (1969), persons respond to this news first with denial and isolation, then anger, then bargaining, followed by depression, and then acceptance. This framework may also be helpful in attending to the responses of members of the family and others close to the terminal illness of a family member or close friend.

THE PROFESSIONAL
AND THE PROCESS OF DYING

The significant roles described in earlier chapters often continue, particularly those dealing with advocacy and communication regarding end-of-life issues. Individuals in the last years of life often complain that they have become invisible: their dependence on care has removed them from the mainstream, resulting in a marginalized existence cut off from those with whom they have ordinarily interacted. One important aspect of advocating and communicating is helping the older person to keep from dropping completely out of sight and to maintain some level of visibility through contact with the outside world. On more than one occasion, professionals have served as spokespersons *for* the dying individual.

Another role of equal importance is when professionals serve as spokespersons *to* the dying individual, providing honest and current information about what is happening to the dying person's body. The sharing of critical information about the patient's well-being and care strategies minimizes the probability of surprises and invites the terminally ill person to become a partner in the program of care.

As each day in the process of dying well seems to become more crucial, professionals may help to bring a level of objectivity and stability to a situation often charged with great emotion by supporting those concerned in dealing with bad news. In addition, they may help the individual and the family advocate for a level of care that emphasizes comfort and that thereby tends to humanize the dying process.

Occasionally professionals, being outsiders to the family, are involved in assisting families to settle disputes. When the wishes of the terminally ill individual conflict with the wishes of family members, particularly regarding end-of-life care, health care professionals, pastors, and others may find themselves needing to mediate the struggle between the desires of those wishing "no extraordinary measures" and those wishing "every possible effort," those wanting to let go and those unwilling to let go. In some instances where the dying person has expressed intent in advance directives, professionals have even found themselves advocating for the patient against the wishes of the family members who would disregard those directives.

Another area of contention may result from new "families" formed in older adulthood. A friend in an extended-care facility developed a very close relationship with another resident in that same facility. Both were retired church workers; he was a widower, she had never married. Having something in common to talk about led to a casual friendship that developed into a very caring, intimate relationship. When she died, his children ignored the grief that he was experiencing and alienated themselves by dismissing their relationship as inconsequential since they weren't married. Professionals are often in a position to alert family members to new realities in an older person's life.

Professionals in this situation also have a responsibility to help family members look beyond the present to that time after the death of the loved one when their own lives will go on. Elderly spouses are sometimes left to fend for themselves. Caregivers who have been consumed with caring for months, if not years, may need support and encouragement to resume living without either the burden or the purposefulness of caregiving. The act of dying resolves all issues for the terminally ill person but leaves issues for those who survive. Professionals and others who support the family at this time may play important roles in aiding them, both in the grieving process and in resuming their other activities, relationships, and responsibilities.

Effectiveness in any of these roles is enhanced by the nature of the relationship a professional builds with the individual and those close to the individual. Those whose contacts are limited to brief functional visits are less likely to be helpful over a broad range of concerns than those who are able to spend time with the older person and those who support the older person, answering questions, offering suggestions, and providing reassurance.

Beneath these important functional areas in which professionals may assist dying persons and those who love them, there is also the need to help persons in the larger and much more nebulous areas of awareness and self-acceptance. It may be difficult for a terminally ill woman to have any sense of self-worth when she knows that there is a large malignant cancer growing with in her, or as Sarton (1978) says, "the hardest thing is knowing that death is there alive inside me" (p. 43). Feelings of self-negation are exacerbated in the further knowledge that she is causing so much concern, expense, and possibly grief and sadness for those she loves. Conversely, those waiting with a dying person may experience feelings of guilt in the knowledge that their confrontation with death is not so immediate and anxiety that their journey through the "valley of the shadow of death" still awaits. Professionals bring varying types of expertise and levels of skill to each situation, but the fundamental need that is shared by all participants is that of accepting themselves as mortal persons.

LANDMARKS AND DEVELOPMENTAL TASKS OF DYING

Ira Byock, a physician who has worked extensively with the dying, has developed a working set of developmental landmarks and tasks. Even accounting for individual differences, Byock (1997b) finds elemental commonalities within the human condition as life ends.

> The end-of-life developmental landmarks and the taskwork that subserve them are intended to represent predictable personal challenges as well as important opportunities of persons as they die. . . . Importantly, within this model one need not sanitize nor glorify the experience of life's end to think of a person as having died well or, similarly, as having achieved a degree of wellness in their dying. Personal development is rarely easy. The touchstone of dying well—the sense of growing individually or together in the midst of dying well—is that the experience is of value and meaningful for the person and their family. (p. 1)

A prescription for dying well is contained in a set of developmental landmarks and tasks for the end of life that provides a framework for thinking about death *developmentally* and with enough precision that an in-depth conversation becomes possible. The framework is divided into landmarks that represent points of accomplishment and tasks necessary to achieve them (Byock, 1997b).

Turning Outward

Byock begins with the assumption that the individual has come to the point where the business of life, the focus of so much life energy until now, is handed over to others. Formal social and legal responsibilities as well as formal relationships in the community are brought to closure. Only a clear sense of the approach of death could bring a person to accomplish this task—to let go of all a person worked so hard to gather, manage, save, and use. In the process of letting go of these formal (i.e., nonfamilial) relationships, there is leave-taking: a time for expressions of regret, forgiveness, thanks, and a saying of good-bye.

For some, the end of formal responsibilities and relationships is a natural element in the larger process of disengagement. For others, it is a great struggle because it signifies, in the words of Henri Nouwen (1985), "the end of our success, our productivity, our fame, or our importance among people" (p. 38), and fails to acknowledge the fullness of the fruit that a life may bear after it is ended.

Turning Inward

When all that is done, the person turns inward, to try to come to a sense of meaning about his or her life. The process is often one of storytelling, to oneself and to others. In this process, failures, wrongs, and things left undone may take on power, but so too may a sense that much good has been done. In this interplay of light and shadow, the individual has to own the good and forgive the bad. This requires an experience of the love of others. Persons can only know themselves truly, forgive themselves convincingly, and love themselves appropriately when they see themselves mirrored in loving faces (Byock, 1996).

Nouwen (1985) claims that it is

> the joy of being the same as others, of belonging to one human family, that allows us to die well. I do not know how I or anyone else could be prepared to die if we were mainly concerned about the trophies we had collected during our best years. The great gift hidden in our dying is the gift of unity with all people. (p. 26)

It may be too much to say that dying is a social event, for often the pain for all involved is too great to foster sociability. Nevertheless, dying well is an act of gratitude, with and for those who have given and reinforced life's meaning.

Now the person is ready to bring to completion relationships with family and friends. Byock sums it up: *"I forgive you; forgive me; thank you; I love you; goodbye"* (1996, p. 246; emphasis added). All these elements speak for themselves. Note, however, that the process of reconciliation is never just a blunt "Forgive me," but rather should be, "I have hurt you. What do you need from me to make it better?"

Letting Go

The final landmarks all have to do with an acceptance that it is okay that one's individual life is coming to an end because there is a transcendent realm. One of May Sarton's characters (1978), on her deathbed, reflects that "we are inextricably woven into a huge web together, and detaching the threads, one by one, is hideously painful. As long as one still feels the tug, one is not ready to die" (p. 183). It is in the surrender to the transcendent, to the unknown, that the final task is completed: One lets go, actively. One wills to surrender. "Here," says Byock (1997b), "little remains of the ego except the volition to surrender" (p. 2).

Each death is unique; yet each death shares commonalities with others that do not diminish an individual's uniqueness. When one is given time for the whole of dying to unfold, these landmarks and developmental tasks will form the agenda for "dying well."

DYING AND RELATIONSHIPS

The kind of dying that all hope for is one that somehow—in the time before the separation of death—brings them close to the ones they love. People long for dying to be as intimate as living, perhaps more so given how vulnerable they will be.

The specifics of dying range from severe suffering to a sense of profound well-being, and the two need not even be separated. There are people whose terminal cancer has given them enormous and intense love in the present moment. Kam was one of these:

> In the last week before Kam died, in his room in an in-hospital hospice, Kam's pain was so intense that he had a morphine pump to use as he needed and as he decided. Mostly, he aimed to balance the level of pain he could tolerate with his desire to be aware and present to his family.

It was midafternoon and the hospice staff had come by with cake and champagne. Kam took some, as did his wife and a friend. Moments later their 20-year-old daughter came in. She sat on her father's bed beside her dad, pushed his morphine pump drip aside so it wouldn't be between them, and shared his cake and champagne with him, sip by sip, nibble by nibble, as Kam's wife watched, gently. Ten years later, the moment is still fresh and real to the friend who was privileged to be there.

Kam's death was too deep for tragedy. Kam died well, and in his dying he, his wife, and his daughter and son all grew together. The experience was of defining value and meaning for Kam and his family. He had handed over his worldly affairs and completed his relationships with the people he had been a pastor to for many years. He had told his stories and shared his wisdom learned as scholar, immigrant, father, husband, citizen, and so on. He acknowledged himself and forgave himself, even for dying so early in the life of his family. He had shared deeply, been grateful, and said good-bye. He accepted his death and turned toward God in silence and willingness to surrender to God's will.

All these acts flowed one into another, and in the end the whole of his life burned in the intensity of one minute, through the dark cold and the empty desolation, into another intensity, a deeper communion—to paraphrase T. S. Eliot (1944). Kam's dying was in love. A desire that one's dying be in love can be a powerful force for being attentive to those most important in life, and it can put little grievances into perspective.

The vision of Kam's dying in community with family and friends is often repeated in situations where time, good relationships, and culture cooperate in what many might idealize as the epitome of dying well. Having spent several weeks with his wife in a hospice, prior to her death, an older gentlemen claimed that "we got to know each other and we grew in love like never before."

Nevertheless, in other situations, the rapid onset of acute illness, inadequate pain management, sudden death, unprepared families, estranged relationships, families at a distance, and a culture that values individualism if not solitude result in situations where dying occurs in isolation. Since various cultures answer the questions surrounding dying and attribute meaning to death in markedly different ways, culturally sanctioned behavior at the time of death is also likely to vary as well. For example, whether death occurs at home, in a hospital, or at an extended-care facility may be a matter of culture as well as economics.

DYING AND MEANING

In a culture that is profoundly secular in its basic orientation, the image of the life course is also profoundly secular, according to Howard Moody (1991):

> What secularity amounts to in practice is that we have no coherent image of the purpose or meaning of old age, nor of the whole of life to which old age is a culmination. . . . Traditional societies have understood death to be the great transition, a momentous turning point in the cycle of our existence on earth. Neither old age nor death have [*sic*] any such significance for the modern world. A telling example of the contrast is that, while modern people want a sudden death, those in traditional societies want time to prepare and ritual practices that reflect that wish. . . . What was once a fate to be avoided—namely, a quick, unanticipated death—becomes for modern man the object of devout (yet secular) prayer. (p. 7)

Even in this cultural milieu, some people have personal attitudes about death born of their religious tradition and commitments. Some can still affirm with Christopher Nugent (1994):

> We do not see the stars save by night. We cannot all reside in nature, but she is still our older resident teacher or, to be more precise, illustrator. And she is rich enough to provide reminders of the miracle of light in the wordless Magnificat of the late October leaves, simultaneously requiem and rainbow. Their very passage is praise. Death is ultimately too deep for tragedy. (p. 103)

People who have actively addressed spiritual issues throughout life may feel, at the end, that their beliefs help them make sense of death and give death meaning. A religious understanding is also likely to incorporate a view of the significance of the suffering that may have preceded death and, perhaps, a view of the afterlife to follow it.

Others who come to the end of life's journey with more questions unanswered than they would like may find in serious illness a time for an important redefinition of the self and may be pushed to rethink what really matters.

> "Why me? Why now? Why this?" The way you come to answer those questions, or "understand what is happening to you," also shapes your spiritual life. . . . The fact that most people find this search to be terribly important and rewarding means that it is worth resisting the temptation to spend all your energy on medical treatment or on relatively unimportant tasks. It is as important to seek space and time for spiritual concerns as it is to seek the right treatment or therapy. (Lynn, Harrold, & the Center to Improve Care of the Dying, 1999, pp. 29-30)

Erik Erikson (1950) writes:

> We all dimly feel that our transient historical identity is the only chance in all eternity to be alive as a somebody in a here and a now. We, therefore, dread the possibility, of which we are most aware when deeply young or very old, that at the end we may find that we have lived the wrong life or not really lived at all. (p. 268)

The task of what Erikson (1950) calls "Ego Integrity vs. Despair" involves finding a sense of meaning in life and death, so that life is accepted as the one and only life that had to be and that life and death convey some world order and spiritual sense, no matter how dearly paid for.

For some, even the absence of any sort of articulated awareness of connections is not of ultimate importance, because they are part of a web of creation that shares spirit. This perspective may be particularly helpful in understanding the meaning-world of those who die in the darkness of dementia. Dorothy Albracht Dougherty and Mary Colgan McNamara (1993) articulate this perspective lyrically:

> For night music is the song of the unconscious, that web of patterns and connections woven in the rich underground world of evolution and history, the collective memory of non-living as well as living beings, that mite of matter through which all of creation shares spirit. Night music melts the separateness of subjectivity and prepares the soul for deep communion. (p. 42)

PREPARATION

In relationships with those most loved there are three "moments" in the journey: dying, the time of death, and the time after death. Each of these can be prepared for.

Preparation for the best possible relationship with those most loved as *one is dying* begins in the present in asking and answering this question:

"If I died now what would be left undone in my relationships with those most important to me?" Death expectancy—the percent of people out of 100 who will die—is 100 percent. This is "a useful number and has its lessons." (Lynch, 1997, p. 5)

Part of the anxiety is not about one's own dying. Some, or even much, of it comes from the thought that those loved most deeply will grieve deeply and suffer much. This could hardly be more real. In all likelihood, those most in love will not die at the same time. People who love deeply grieve deeply. But grief can end and life can be full again. Perhaps the truth is that the most telling glimpse into death's harsh finality comes through the loving eyes of the beloved. That is why some grieve now with anticipatory grief for those closest to them who will bear, in love, the burdens of grief.

It is not only grief they will carry, but the burden of making sure that the one who has died is not forgotten. It is a constancy in intimacy of soul and heart that is asked for—being held in heart and mind in loving memory when most others have forgotten.

Preparation for the best possible relationship with those most loved *when one dies* is made possible when issues have been talked through and preparations made for the "how" of care at the time of death. Advance directives and medical power of attorney are only part of this. More central to relationships is a clear, common set of convictions about what death is and how the journey of life should end. A final illness raises important questions about the amount of intervention to be pursued, about when to discontinue efforts to keep the patient alive, about when to let go. This is not something easily come to, nor something that is accomplished once for all. Clear understanding and common conviction help both the patient and those who care about the patient address their own ambivalence about death and help them to avoiding panicking in a moment of distress.

It is important that much attention be given to those aspects of dying that are addressed in advance directives and that involve medical personnel and systems. Paramount may be the question of place. Most Americans want to die at home, familiar and comfortable and safe. But few die without requiring a great deal of assistance with bathing, feeding, and toileting, to say nothing of the medications that may need to be administered, and the medical care provided. Often those available to provide these services are themselves burdened with responsibility, anxiety, and grief. Dying at home may be the result of conscious choices or economic default, but in either case, plans must include the gathering of a cadre of caregivers adequate to the need.

The increasing availability of hospice also addresses the question of place. Hospice services come in various types: some provide services to the dying in their homes; others are attached to hospitals and have a hospital-like setting; and still others are like a home away from home. Hospice personnel have special experience alleviating pain and providing comfort to the dying.

There are also other issues that merit consideration. Are there particular persons whom the dying individual wishes to have present? Are there particular elements to be introduced into the environment to aid in the transition? One very proper lady wanted her daughter to promise that she would make certain her hair was combed, and that she was wearing her favorite perfume. A friend let her family know that she wished to die to the music of Mahler's Second Symphony. Believing in its soothing power, a program is being developed in various locations to provide the live music of harps and voices at bedside to relieve the mental and physical pain of patients facing the end of life.

There is doubtless a fine line between micromanaging death and providing a setting for the terminally ill person to die in peace and comfort. But the entire process of preparation may more importantly provide the occasion for frank conversation about end-of-life plans and issues, increasing comfort with confronting the death of a loved one as well as one's own death, and increasing support for the terminally ill person, knowing that he or she does not confront this mystery alone.

The preceding paragraphs describe something of a partnership in preparation in which both terminally ill persons and those who love them share in the planning. But with some frequency this is not possible because the dying persons suffer confusion, forgetfulness, hallucinations, or dementia, making their participation in such planning impossible. Since these consciousness-altering states may befall any person, it seems obvious that the partnership in planning is wisely commenced long before diagnoses of terminal illness occur.

Preparation for the best possible relationship with those most loved *after death* comes about when there are clear decisions, shared and written, about what is to happen. It is important to be particularly attentive in these preparations to the fact that the burden of grief is on those who are left. Their feelings and sensitivities need to be paramount.

In *The Undertaking: Life Studies from the Dismal Trade,* Thomas Lynch (1997) puts it bluntly and forcefully:

> Any damage or decency we do accrues to the living, to whom your death happens, if it really happens to anyone. The living have to live with it. You don't. Theirs is the grief or gladness your death brings. Theirs is the loss or gain of it. Theirs is the pain and the pleasure of memory. Theirs is the invoice for services rendered and theirs is the check in the mail for its payment. (p. 7)

In making last wishes clear, attention must be given to the rituals that bring initial closure to death. For example, someone may wish to have his remains cremated. It can't matter to him, but it may be dreadfully important to those who love this person that his body is present for wake and funeral so that they can bring closure in a way with which they are comfortable. And vice versa—many who find viewing a body offensive may be brought to do so only by the wishes of the deceased.

Relationships that include attention to these realities and open conversation about them are intimate, threatening, easily avoided, but key to healthy living. Make no mistake—it can be personally threatening. Writing one's obituary, deciding on cremation or burial, contemplating a wake, planning a funeral—all these are a sort of final "examination of conscience," the last, stark weighing in, the non-sugar-coated version of a person. It is only in a gaze of love that it is possible to let go of these fears and judge oneself gracefully. All the more reason to nourish now what will be of final importance.

THE NEED TO IMPROVE CARE
AT THE END OF LIFE

The likelihood of experiencing the kind of death one chooses has implication for institutions and communities as well as families, clinicians, benefits managers and purchasers, citizens, and policymakers. What most will experience at the end of life depends upon community commitment and action. "Dying well, to many, means control over choices to be made as we die. We fear dying in pain; we fear that too much will be done to keep us alive, or we fear that not enough will be done" (Moyers, 2000, p. 12).

There are a number of coalitions being formed to effect change. For example, Americans for Better Care of the Dying (ABCD) (2000) is an organization based in Washington, DC, that is dedicated to ensuring that all Americans can count on good end-of-life care. Their goals are to build momentum for reform, to explore new methods and systems for delivering care, and to shape public policy through evidence-based understanding. They aim to accomplish these goals by focusing their efforts on fundamental reforms, such as improved pain management, better financial reimbursement systems, enhanced continuity of care, support for family caregivers, and changes in public policy. In addition to the work of Moyers (2000) and Americans for Better Care of the Dying (2000), other online resources addressing end-of-life issues include Growth House (n.d.), National Hospice and Palliative Care Organization (2003), Last Acts (n.d.), and Partnership for Caring (2003).

Americans for Better Care of the Dying (2000) list seven promises that need to be made to all citizens, drawn from Lynn, Schuster, and Kabcenell's *Improving Care at the End of Life* (2000). A moment's reflection makes it evident that society is far from fulfilling these promises, no matter how fundamental they are to all human lives.

1. You will have the best of medical treatment, aiming to prevent exacerbation, improve function and survival, and ensure comfort.
2. You will never have to endure overwhelming pain, shortness of breath, or other symptoms.
3. Your care will be continuous, comprehensive, and coordinated.

4. You and your family will be prepared for everything that is likely to happen in the course of your illness.
5. Your wishes will be sought and respected, and followed whenever possible.
6. We will help you to consider your personal and financial resources and we will respect your choices about their use.
7. We will do all we can to see that you and your family will have the opportunity to make the best of every day.

This consideration of dying has moved from a personal consideration of death out into the world of systems, politics, and community action. Accounts of how persons die and policies allowing certain medical practices that facilitate comfortable deaths have become newsworthy and highly politicized. That may seem curious or even inappropriate. But the reality of the situation and the witness of people like Ira Byock, MD, and Bill Moyers make it clear that the personal ability to die as one chooses is not a solitary pursuit. Public policy shapes the care of all who are dying. Models of change that deal with issues of dying in more human ways are desperately needed.

Thomas Cole (1992), the author of *The Journey of Life,* writes what we may take as a suitable epitaph for this consideration of dying—words worth remembering and living by:

Aging is a moral and spiritual frontier because its unknowns, terrors, and mysteries cannot be successfully crossed without humility and self-knowledge, without love and compassion, without acceptance of physical decline and mortality and a sense of the sacred. (p. 243)

Epilogue

Prevailing:
A Challenge and a Vision

This book has been written for professionals and other helpers who advise older persons already on the way or those looking ahead, and who provide personal support as well as professional skill. These professionals and other helpers are key in helping to frame issues and discover solutions, listening to the accounts of triumph as well as travail, moving through the stability and change inherent in the periods, and thereby shaping the journey. The role of the professional and others in their relationship with the older person is twofold. First, they journey as dependable companions; and second, at every age they also anticipate their own journey, seeing themselves in the faces of clients, patients, parishioners, and family members. Perhaps more important even than the skills that professionals bring to the "Journey Called Aging" is the vision of what is possible—that people can thrive throughout the whole of life, and that all life is holy.

Whether journeying with or simply looking ahead, the reader has been led through the highs and lows, the calms and the storms, the obstacles and the opportunities of the journey, to understand the particular dynamics of older adulthood, and to see the various components against the background of the whole. In the process, the paradox described by Florida Scott-Maxwell (1968) in her eighty-fifth year becomes clear:

We who are old know that age is more than a disability. It is an intense and varied experience, almost beyond our capacity at

A Journey Called Aging: Challenges and Opportunities in Older Adulthood
© 2007 by The Haworth Press, Taylor & Francis Group. All rights reserved.
doi:10.1300/5915_10

times, but something to be carried high. If it is a long defeat it is also a victory, meaningful for the initiates of time, if not for those who have come less far. (p. 5)

The book was written within a cultural context that glamorizes youth and denies the presence of aging and death. Euphemisms cloak the realities of the latter years of life, and death is hidden in silence. Social programs address some of the problems of the neediest of aging citizens without addressing more broadly the challenges and opportunities inherent in these years. Medical advances, in addressing what were often fatal illnesses in middle age, have increased the numbers of persons who live to an advanced age. Those advances, together with accounts of research examining strategies to increase human longevity, feed the illusion that science and technology may eliminate the problems of aging and death altogether. To succumb to this illusory hope for the future is to refuse to accept the reality of aging and death in the present.

When William Faulkner received the Nobel Prize for Literature, he gave a strong endorsement for the triumph of the human spirit. Faulkner (1968) said, "I believe that man will not merely endure: he will prevail" [*text not edited for gender inclusiveness*] (p. 5). Prevailing in older adulthood does not mean being excused from losses or pain, nor of being eased out of life so as not to face the deep ruts in the journey. Prevailing is facing it all, staring it down, growing into a better person for it, and moving ahead until the end.

In this book there have been stories of prevailing. They were not simply the happy tales of the good life, although such are defining moments in late life for some. They included voices that are inexhaustible not because of health and wealth and strength, but because they are the voices of people who had developed, in the words of T. R. Cole (1994) (quoting Max Weber), a "trained relentlessness in viewing the realities of life and the ability to face such realities and measure up to them inwardly" (p. 1).

Examples of prevailing occur among family members, friends, professional clients, and others in the journey from retiring to dying. Some of these contemporaries and peers traverse life stages with great panache and verve, confronting challenges, taking advantage of every opportunity for personal growth, and prevailing over losses and difficulties. Some maintain high levels of purpose and productivity into advanced years. But some seem overwhelmed by the years and all that they bring: courage is lost, ideals are abandoned, a stubborn and admittedly illogical resistance to change grips the soul, the hardships of illness and poverty seem to crush the spirit.

Perhaps more important even than the skills that professionals bring to the "Journey Called Aging" is the vision of what is possible and what is necessary. This book has endeavored to inform and shape that vision. It is a vision of prevailing, as every loss becomes an opportunity for growth. Those who journey together as adults and as older adults both challenge and support one another as they negotiate the vagaries and the sometimes difficult times they confront. In a variety of substantial and meaningful ways in the intense and varied experience of growing old, singularly and together, let a spirit capable of growing and enduring be kindled and released so that all may prevail.

References

Administration on Aging (1997). *National Elder Abuse Incidence Study.* Retrieved June 2, 2006, from http://www.aoa.eldfam/Elder_Rights/Elder_Abuse/Abuse Report_Full.pdf.

Alliance for Aging Research (n.d.). *Ageism: How Healthcare Fails the Elderly.* Washington, DC: Alliance for Aging Research. Retrieved May 30, 2006, from http://www.agingresearch.org/brochures/ageism/index.cfm.

American Psychological Association (2003, September). *Facts About Depression in Older Adults.* APA Online. Retrieved September 3, 2004, from http://www.apa.org/ppo/issues/olderdepressfact.html.

American Psychological Association (2004, May-June). Guidelines for psychological practice with older adults. *American Psychologist, 59*(4), 236-260.

Americans for Better Care of the Dying (2000). Washington, DC. Retrieved December 26, 2003, from www.abcd-caring.org.

Arias, E., Anderson, R.N., Kung, H.C., Murphy, S.L., & Kochanek, K.D. (2003, September 18). *Deaths: Final Data for 2001* (National Vital Statistics Reports), *52*, Tables 4, 7. Washington, DC: U.S. Department of Health and Human Services, Centers for Disease Control and Prevention.

Aschenbaum, W.A., & Bengston, V.L. (1994). Re-engaging the disengagement theory of aging: On the history and assessment of theory development in gerontology. *The Gerontologist, 34*(6), 756-763.

Atchley, R.C. (1976). *The Sociology of Retirement.* New York: Halsted.

Atchley, R.C. (1983). *Aging: Continuity and Change.* Belmont, CA: Wadsworth.

Attig, T. (2001). Relearning the World: Making and Finding Meanings. In R.A. Neimeyer (Ed.), *Meaning Reconstruction and the Experience of Loss* (pp. 33-54). Washington, DC: American Psychological Association.

Baltes, M.M., & Lang, F.R. (1997, September). Everyday functioning and successful aging: The impact of resources. *Psychology and Aging, 12*(3), 433-443.

Baltes, P.B., & Baltes, M.M. (1990). Psychological Perspectives on Successful Aging: The Model of Selective Optimization with Compensation. In P.B. Baltes & M.M. Baltes (Eds.), *Successful Aging: Perspectives from the Behavioral Sciences* (pp. 1-27). Cambridge: Press Syndicate of the University of Cambridge.

Baltes, P.B., & Baltes, M.M. (1998, Spring). Savoir vivre in old age: How to master the shifting balance between gains and losses. *National Forum, 78*(2), 13-18.

Basler, B. (2006, February). Assisted living: 10 great ideas. *AARP Bulletin,* 16-24.

Bassuk, S.S., Glass, T.A., & Berkman, L.F. (1999). Social disengagement and incident cognitive decline in community-dwelling elderly persons. *Annals of Internal Medicine, 131,* 165-173. Retrieved December 5, 2003, from http://www.annals.org.

Belgrave, L.L., Wykle, M.L., & Choi, J.M. (1993). Health, double jeopardy, and culture: The use of institutionalization by African Americans. *The Gerontologist, 33*(3), 379-385.

Berger, R.M., & Kelly, J.J. (2000). What Are Older Gay Men Like? An Impossible Question? In D.C. Kimmel & D.L. Martin (Eds.), *Midlife and Aging in Gay America* (pp. 55-64). Binghamton, NY: The Haworth Press.

Bernasek, A. (2006, January 29). The golden years: Travels, hobbies and new job, too. *New York Times,* Section 3, 5. Retrieved April 18, 2006, from http://select.nytimes.com/gst/abstract.html?res=F30D1FFB3A5B0C7A8EDDA80894DE404482.

Bernstein, L., & Schwartz, S. (1989). *Mass: A Theatre Piece of Singers, Players, and Dancers.* New York: Boosey and Hawkes (originally published 1971).

Bolen, J.S. (1996). *Close to the Bone: Life-Threatening Illness and the Search for Meaning.* New York: Simon and Schuster.

Boyce, A., Wethington, E., & Moen, P. (2003). Continuity and Change in Subjective Well-Being. In J.A. Krout & E. Wethington (Eds.), *Residential Choices and Experiences of Older Adults: Pathways to Life Quality* (pp. 177-196). New York: Springer.

Boyd, M., with a foreword by Martin E. Marty (2001). *Simple Grace: A Mentor's Guide to Growing Older.* Louisville, KY: Westminster John Knox.

Brandstädter, J., & Baltes-Götz, B. (1990). Personal Control Over Development and Quality of Life Perspectives in Adulthood. In P.B. Baltes & M.M. Baltes (Eds.), *Successful Aging: Perspectives from the Behavioral Sciences* (pp. 197-224). Cambridge: Press Syndicate of the University of Cambridge.

Bridges, W. (1980). *Transitions: Making Sense of Life's Changes.* Reading, MA: Addison-Wesley.

Brim, G. (1988, September). Losing and winning. *Psychology Today, 22*(9), 48-52.

Brown, L.B., Alley, G.R., Sorosy, S., Quarto, G., & Look, T. (2000). Gay Men: Aging Well! In D.C. Kimmel & D.L. Martin (Eds.), *Midlife and Aging in Gay America* (pp. 41-54). Binghamton, NY: The Haworth Press.

Brown, S.L., Nesse, R.M., Vinokur, A.D., & Smith, D.M. (2003, July). Providing social support may be more beneficial than receiving it: Results from a prospective study of mortality. *Psychological Science, 14*(4), 320-327.

Buber, M. (1937). *I and Thou* (R.G. Smith, trans.). New York: Charles Scribner's Sons.

Buechner, F. (1973). *Wishful Thinking.* New York: Harper.

Byock, I. (1996, May). The nature of suffering and the nature of opportunity at the end of life. *Clinics in Geriatric Medicine, 12*(2), 237-252.

Byock, I. (1997a). *Dying Well: Peace and Possibilities at the End of Life.* New York: Riverhead.

Byock, I. (1997b). *Dying Well: Working Set of Landmarks and Developmental Taskwork.* Retrieved December 26, 2003, from http://www.dyingwell.com/landmarks.htm.

Campbell, J. (1988). *The Power of Myth*. New York: Doubleday.

Carbonell, J.G. (2003, May 20). *Baby Boomers at the Gate: Enhancing Independence Through Innovation and Technology*. Testimony Given to Senate Special Committee on Aging. Washington, DC. Retrieved July 21, 2003, from http://aging.senate.gov/index.cfm?Fuseaction=Hearings.Testimony&HearingID=19&WitnessID=69.

Carnahan, J. (2002, February 6). Opening Statement. *Women and Aging: Bearing the Burden of Long-Term Care*. Joint Hearing of the Senate Special Committee on Aging and the Subcommittee on Aging. Senate Committee on Health, Education, Labor, and Pensions, 107th Cong., 2nd Session. Retrieved May 31, 2006, from http://www.senate.gov/Hearings/2002_02_06/Carnahan.pdf.

Carstensen, L.L. (2001). Selectivity Theory: Social Activity in Life-Span Context. In A.J. Walker, M. Manoogian-O'Dell, L.A. McGraw, & D.L.G. White (Eds.), *Families in Later Life: Connections and Transitions* (pp. 265-275). Thousand Oaks, CA: Pine Forge.

Carter, J. (1998). *The Virtues of Aging*. New York: Ballantine.

Carter, J. (2001). *An Hour Before Daylight*. New York: Simon and Schuster.

Cavafy, C.P. (1995). Ithaka. In E. Keeley (Ed.), *The Essential Cavafy*. New York: Ecco.

CBSNews.com (2002, July 30). Older Americans "shacking up" more. Washington, DC: CBS News. Retrieved September 1, 2002, from http://www.cbsnews.com/stories/2002/07/03/national/main516814.shtml.

Centers for Disease Control and Prevention (1998). AIDS among persons aged greater than or equal to 50 years—United States, 1991-1996. *Morbidity and Mortality Weekly Report, 47*(2), 21-27.

Centers for Disease Control and Prevention (2001a). *Basic Statistics. Divisions of HIV/AIDS Prevention*. Atlanta, GA: Department of Health and Human Services, Public Health Service. Retrieved December 26, 2003, from http://www.cdc.gov/his/stats.htm.

Centers for Disease Control and Prevention (2001b). *HIV/AIDS Surveillance Report, 13*, Table 7. Atlanta, GA: Department of Health and Human Services, Public Health Service.

Centers for Disease Control and Prevention (2003). Aids cases in adolescents and adults, by age—United States, 1994-2000. *HIV/AIDS Surveillance Supplemental Report, 9*, Table 10. Atlanta, GA: Department of Health and Human Services, Public Health Service.

Centers for Medicare and Medicaid Services (2005). *Medicare Compare*. Baltimore, MD: U.S. Dept. of Health and Human Services. Retrieved June 12, 2006, from http://www.Medicare.gov/NHCompare.

Charles, S.T., Mather, M., & Carstensen, L.L. (2003). Aging and emotional memory: The forgettable nature of negative images for older adults. *Journal of Experimental Psychology General, 132*(2), 310-324.

Clark, D. (2002, April 13). Between hope and acceptance: The medicalisation of dying. *BMJ Journal, 324*, 905-907. Retrieved September 1, 2002, from http://www.BMJ.com.

Clark, M., & Anderson, B. (1967). *Culture and Aging*. Springfield, IL: Thomas.

Clendenen, A. (2002, April). She's circling the drain. *Second Opinion,* 110.

Cohen, D. (2003, July 28). Depression and Violent Deaths in Older Americans: An Emergent Public Mental Health Challenge. *Senior Depression: Life-Saving Mental Health Treatments for Older Americans.* Hearing before the Senate Special Committee on Aging, 108th Cong., 1st Session, 5.

Cohler, B.J. (1993). Aging, Morale, and Meaning: The Nexus of Narrative. In T.R. Cole, W.A. Achenbaum, P.L. Jakobi, & R. Kastenbaum (Eds.), *Voices and Visions of Aging: Toward a Critical Gerontology* (pp. 107-133). New York: Springer.

Cole, C. (1986, March). Developmental tasks affecting the marital relationship in later life. *American Behavior Scientist, 29*(4), 389-403.

Cole, T.R. (1992). *The Journey of Life: A Cultural History of Aging in America.* New York: Cambridge.

Cole, T.R. (1994, Spring). Editorial. *Aging and the Human Spirit, 4*(1), 1.

Cole, T.R. (1997). What Have We "Made" of Aging? In M. Freedman (Ed.), *Critical Issues in Aging, No. 1: An Annual Magazine of the American Society on Aging, 1,* 59-60.

Cristofer, M. (1977). *The Shadow Box: A Drama in Two Acts.* New York: Samuel French.

Cumming, E., & Henry, W.C. (1961). *Growing Old: The Process of Disengagement.* New York: Basic Books.

Cusack, S.A., & Thompson, W.J.A. (1999). *Leadership for Older Adults. Aging with Purpose and Passion.* Philadelphia: Taylor and Francis.

DeBeauvoir, S. (1972). *The Coming of Age* (P. O'Brian, trans.). New York: Putnam's.

Didion, J. (2005). *The Year of Magical Thinking.* New York: Knopf.

Dougherty, D.A., & McNamara, M.C. (1993). *Out of the Skin, Into the Soul: The Art of Aging.* San Diego, CA: LuraMedia.

Dresang, J. (2005, March 7). At 85, factory worker still setting the pace. *Milwaukee Journal Sentinel,* 1A, 13A.

Dressel, P. (Ed.). (1996). Grandparenting at century's end. *Generations, 20,* 80.

Egan, P. (1996, September). Side Glances. Rest homes for the 21st century. *Road and Track, 48*(1), 322-336.

Elderly show their emotional know-how (1999). *Science News, 155,* 374.

Eliot, T.S. (1994). East Coker (lines 205-207). *Four Quartets.* London: Faber and Faber.

Erikson, E. (1950). *Childhood and Society.* New York: Norton.

Erikson, J. (1997). New Chapters in the Ninth Stage. In J. Erikson (Ed.), *The Life Cycle Completed: Extended Version.* New York: Norton (original version, Erik Erikson, 1982).

Fahey, C.J., & Holstein, M. (1993). Toward a Philosophy of the Third Age. In T.R. Cole, W.A. Ashenbaum, P.O. Jakobi, & R. Kastenbaum (Eds.), *Voices and Visions of Aging: Toward a Critical Gerontology* (pp. 241-256). New York: Springer.

Faulkner, W. (1996). *Essays, Speeches, and Public Letters.* New York: Random House.

Fein, E. (1994, August 9). "Card game is helping 6 friends trump age." *New York Times,* A16.

Field, D. (1997). Looking back, what period of life brought you the most satisfaction. *International Journal of Aging and Human Development, 45*(3), 169-194.

Fisher, J.C. (1986). Participation in educational activities by active older adults. *Adult Education Quarterly, 36*(4), 138-146.

Fisher, J.C. (1993). A framework for describing developmental change among older adults. *Adult Education Quarterly, 43*(2), 76-89.

Fisher, J.C. (1998). Major Streams of Research Probing Older Adult Learning. In J.C. Fisher and M.A. Wolf (Eds.), *Using Learning to Meet the Challenges of Older Adulthood* (No. 77 in New Directions for Adult and Continuing Education) (pp. 27-40). San Francisco: Jossey-Bass.

Flacks, R. (1988). *Making History.* New York: Columbia.

Freund, A.M., & Baltes, P.B. (2002). Life-management strategies of selection, optimization, and compensation: Measurement by self-report and construct validity. *Journal of Personality and Social Psychology, 82*(4), 642-662.

Frost, R. (1930). *Complete Poems.* London: Henry Holt.

Fry, P.S. (2001, December). Predictors of health-related quality of life perspectives, self-esteem, and life satisfactions of older adults following spousal loss. *The Gerontologist, 41*(6), 787-798.

Gendell, M. (2000). Trends in retirement age in four countries, 1965-1995. *Monthly Labor Review.* Bethesda, MD: Congressional Information Service, Inc.

Gergen, K., & Gergen, M. (2002, February 27). *The Positive Aging Newsletter.* Retrieved May 26, 2006, from http://taosinstitute.net/resources/pa11.html.

Gerzon, M. (1992). *Coming Into Our Own: Understanding the Adult Metamorphosis.* New York: Delacorte.

Gilligan, C. (1982). *In a Different Voice.* Cambridge, MA: Harvard University.

Godwin, G. (1999). *Evensong.* New York: Random House.

Gray, R.H. (1986). *Survival of the Spirit: My Detour In and Out of a Retirement Home.* Atlanta, GA: John Knox.

Groger, L., Mayberry, P.S., Straker, J.K., & Mehdizadeh, S. (1997). *African-American Elders' Long-Term Care Preferences and Choices* (Administration on Aging No. 90-AR-2034). Washington, DC: U.S. Department of Health and Human Services. Retrieved May 30, 2006, from www.cas.muohio.edu/scripps/pdf/AfrAmPreferences.pdf.

Growth House (n.d.). Retrieved December 26, 2003, from http://www.growth house.org.

Gubrium, J.F. (1993). Voice and Context in a New Gerontology. In T.R. Cole, W.A. Achenbaum, P.L. Jakobi, & R. Kastenbaum (Eds.), *Voices and Visions of Aging: Toward a Critical Gerontology* (pp. 46-63). New York: Springer.

Haan, M.N. (1999). Can social engagement prevent cognitive decline in old age? *Annals of Internal Medicine, 131,* 220-221. Retrieved December 5, 2003, from http://www.annals.org.

Hagman, G. (2001). Beyond Decathexis: Toward a New Psychoanalytic Understanding and Treatment of Mourning. In Robert A. Neimeyer (Ed.), *Meaning Reconstruction and the Experience of Loss* (pp. 13-32). Washington, DC: American Psychological Association.

Hale, C. (2000, October). My father lost and found. *Health,* 136-138, 172.

Hall, E. (1983, June). A conversation with Erik Erikson. *Psychology Today, 17*(6), 22-30.

Hargrave, T. (1994). *Families and Forgiveness: Healing Wounds in the Intergenerational Family.* New York: Brunner/Mazel.

Havighurst, R. (1952). *Developmental Tasks and Education.* New York: McKay.

Havighurst, R.J., Cavan, R., Burgess, W.E., & Goldhammer, H. (1949). *Personal Adjustment in Old Age.* Chicago: Science Research Associates.

He, W., Sengupta, M., Velkoff, V.A., & DeBarros, K.A. (2005). *65+ in the United States, 2005* (U.S. Census Bureau Current Publications Reports, P23-209). Washington, DC: U.S. Government Printing Office.

Heidrich, S.M. (1993). The relationship between physical health and psychological well-being in elderly women: A developmental perspective. *Research in Nursing & Health, 16,* 123-130.

Heidrich, S.M. (1994, October). The self, health, and depression in elderly women. *Western Journal of Nursing Research, 16*(5), 544-555.

Heilbrun, C. (1997). *The Last Gift of Time: Life Beyond Sixty.* New York: Dial.

Hetzel, L., & Smith, A. (2001). *The 65 Years and Over Population: 2000* (Census 2000 Brief C2KBR/01-10). Washington, DC: U.S. Census Bureau, U.S. Department of Commerce. Retrieved May 25, 2006, from http://www.census.gov/prod/2001pubs/c2kbr01-10.pdf.

Howard, D.L., Sloane, P.D., Zimmerman, S., Eckert, J.K., Walsh, J.F., Buie, V.C. et. al. (2002, August). Distribution of African Americans in residential care/assisted living and nursing homes: More evidence of racial disparity. *American Journal of Public Health, 92*(8), 1272-1277.

Hoyert, D.L., Arias, E., Smith, B.L., Murphy, S.L., & Kochanek, K.D. (2001, September 21). Deaths: Final data for 1999. *National Vital Statistics Reports, 49*(8). Washington, DC: U.S. Department of Health and Human Services Centers for Disease Control and Prevention.

Hull, J. (2000). *Losing Julia.* New York: Delacorte.

Hultsch, D.V., & Deutsch, F. (1981). *Adult Development and Aging: A Life-Span Perspective.* New York: McGraw-Hill.

Huyck, M.H., & Hoyer, W.J. (1982). *Adult Development and Aging.* Belmont, CA: Wadsworth.

Illich, I. (1976). *Limits to Medicine.* London: Marion Boyars.

Independent Sector (1999). *Giving and Volunteering in the United States, 1999.* Washington, DC.

Jarvis, P. (1989). Retirement: An incomplete ritual. *Journal of Educational Gerontology, 4*(2), 79-84.

Johns Hopkins Magazine, September 1993, p. 28.

Johnson, C.L. (1995). Cultural Diversity in the Late-Life Family. In R. Blieszner & V.H. Bedford (Eds.), *Handbook of Aging and the Family* (pp. 307-331). Westport, CT: Greenwood.

Johnson, C.L. (1995, Autumn). Determinants of adaptation of older old black Americans. *Journal of Aging Studies, 9*(3), 231-244.

Johnson, C.L. (2000). Perspectives on American kinship in the later 1990s. *Journal of Marriage & Family, 62*(3), 623-639.

Johnson, C.L., & Barer, B.M. (1997). *Life Beyond 85 Years: The Aura of Survivorship*. Springfield, IL: Springer.

Johnson, R.W., & Wiener, J.M. (2006). A Profile of Frail Older Americans and Their Caregivers. *The Retirement Project* (Occasional Paper Number 8). Washington, DC: Urban Institute. Retrieved May 15, 2006, from http://www.urban.org/publications/311254.html.

Jung, C. (1933). *Modern Man in Search of a Soul*. New York: Harcourt Brace.

Kahn, R.L. (1994). Social Support: Content, Causes, and Consequences. In R.P. Abeles, H.C. Gift, & M.G. Ory (Eds.), *Aging and Quality of Life* (pp. 163-184). New York: Springer.

Kastenbaum, R. (1993). Encrusted Elders: Arizona and the Political Spirit of Postmodern Aging. In T.R. Cole, W.A. Achenbaum, P.L. Jakobi, & R. Kastenbaum (Eds.), *Voices and Visions of Aging: Toward a Critical Gerontology* (pp. 160-183). New York: Springer.

Kaufman, S.R. (1986). *The Ageless Self: Sources of Meaning in Late Life*. Madison, WI: University of Wisconsin.

Kaufman, S.R. (1998, December). Intensive care, old age, and the problem of death in America. *The Gerontologist, 38*(6), 715-725.

Kidder, T. (1993). *Old Friends*. Boston: Houghton Mifflin.

Kiyak, H.A., & Hooyman, N.R. (1994). Minority and Socioeconomic Status: Impact on Quality of Life in Aging. In R.P. Abeles, H.C. Gift, & M.G. Ory (Eds.), *Aging and Quality of Life* (pp. 295-315). New York: Springer.

Klaus, C.H. (1999). *Taking Retirement: A Beginner's Diary*. Boston: Beacon.

Kreitlow, B., & Kreitlow, D. (1997). *Creative Planning for the Second Half of Life*. Duluth, MN: Whole Person Associates.

Kreitlow, D.J., & Kreitlow, B.W. (1989). Careers after 60: Choices in retirement. *Adult Learning, 1*(5), 10-13.

Krout, J.A., & Pillemer, K. (2003). Lessons for Providers and Consumers. In J.A. Krout & E. Withington (Eds.), *Residential Choices and Experiences of Older Adults: Pathways to Life Quality* (pp. 197-210). New York: Springer.

Krout, J.A., & Wethington, E. (2003). Introduction. In J.A. Krout & E. Wethington, (Eds.), *Residential Choices and Experiences of Older Adults: Pathways to Life Quality* (pp. 3-26). New York: Springer.

Kübler-Ross, E. (1969). *On Death and Dying: What the Dying Have to Teach Doctors, Nurses, Clergy and Their Own Families*. New York: Macmillan.

Kunitz, S. (2000). *The Layers: Collected Poems*. New York: Norton.

Last Acts (n.d.). Retrieved December 26, 2003, from http://www.lastacts.org.

Lee, R.D. (2003, July 15). Rethinking the evolutionary theory of aging: Transfers, not births, shape senescence in social species. *New York Times*, F3.

Levinson, D.J. (1986). A conception of adult development. *American Psychologist, 41*(1), 3-13.

Levinson, D.J., Darrow, C.N., Klein, E.B., Levinson, M.H., & McKee, B. (1978). *The Seasons of a Man's Life*. New York: Ballantine.

Levinson, D.J., & Levinson, J.D. (1996). *The Seasons of a Woman's Life*. New York: Knopf.

Lewis, C.S. (1961). *A Grief Observed*. Minneapolis, MN: Seabury.

Luckey, I. (1994, February). African American elders: The support network of generational kin. *Families in Society, 75*(2), 82-89.

Lusardi, A., & Mitchell, O.S. (2005, December). *Financial Literacy and Planning: Implications for Retirement Wellbeing.* Ann Arbor, MI: University of Michigan Retirement Research Center. Retrieved February 6, 2006, from http://www.mrrc.isr.umich.edu/publications/papers/pdf/wp108.pdf.

Lustbader, W. (2001). *What's Worth Knowing.* New York: Tarcher/Putnam.

Lynch, T. (1997). *The Undertaking: Life Studies from the Dismal Trade.* New York: Penguin.

Lynn, J., Harrold, J., & the Center to Improve Care of the Dying (1999). *Handbook for Mortals: Guidance for People Facing Serious Illness.* New York: Oxford.

Lynn, J., Schuster, J.L., & Kabcenell, A. (2000). *Improving Care for the End of Life.* New York: Oxford.

MacBean, E.C., & Simmons, H.C. (2006). *Thriving Beyond Midlife.* Richmond, VA: Institute for Integral Retirement Planning.

MacKinlay, E. (2001). The spiritual dimension of caring: Applying a model for spiritual tasks of ageing. *Journal of Religious Gerontology, 12*(3/4), 151-166.

Manheimer, R.J., Snodgrass, D.D., & Moskow-McKenzie, D. (1995). *Older Adult Education: A Guide to Research, Programs, and Policies.* Westport, CT: Greenwood Press.

Manton, K.G., & Gu, X.L. (2001, May). Changes in the prevalence of chronic disability in the United States black and nonblack population above age 65 from 1982 to 1999. *Proceedings of the National Academy of Science, 98*(11), 6354-6359.

Maslow, A.H. (1971). *The Farther Reaches of Human Nature.* New York: Viking.

McClusky, H.Y. (1971). *Education: Background Paper for 1971 White House Conference on Aging.* Washington, DC: White House Conference on Aging.

McCullough, L.B. (1993). Arrested Aging: The Power of the Past to Make Us Aged and Old. In T.R. Cole, W.A. Achenbaum, P.L. Jakobi, & R. Kastenbaum (Eds.), *Voices and Visions of Aging: Toward a Critical Gerontology* (pp. 184-204). New York: Springer.

Merkin, D. (2004, May 2). Keeping the forces of decrepitude at bay. *The New York Times Magazine,* 64-67, 96, 101-102.

Merriam, S.B. (1983). *Themes of Adulthood Through Literature.* New York: Teacher's College.

Metropolitan Diary (1998, March 2). *New York Times,* A18.

Moody, H.R. (1986). The Meaning of Life and the Meaning of Old Age. In T.R. Cole and S.A. Gadow (Eds.), *What Does It Mean to Grow Old? Reflections from the Humanities* (pp. 11-40). Durham, NC: Duke.

Moody, H.R. (1991, Spring). From "Sacred and contemporary concepts of lifespan development." *Aging and the Human Spirit, 1*(1), 7.

Moody, H.R. (2003, August 15). Assisted Suicide: Loss of Faith in Medical Care. *The Soul of Bioethics.* New York: International Longevity Center—USA.

Moss, B.F., & Schwebel, A.I. (1993, January). Defining intimacy in romantic relationships. *Family Relations, 42*(1), 31-37.

Moyers, B. (2000). *On Our Own Terms: Moyers on Dying in America: Leadership Guide.* New York: Public Affairs Television. Retrieved June 2, 2006, from http://www-tc.pbs.org/wnet/onourownterms/community/pdf/discussionguide.pdf?mii=1.

Murray, C.J.L., Michaud, C.M., McKenna, M., & Marks, J. (1998). *US Patterns of Mortality by County and Race: 1965-1994.* Cambridge, MA: Harvard Center for Population and Development Studies.

Myerhoff, B. (1978). *Number Our Days.* New York: Dutton.

Nagurney, A.J., Reich, J.W., & Newsom, J.T. (2004). Gender moderates the effects of independence and dependence desires during the social support process. *Psychology and Aging, 19*(1), 215-218.

National Center for Education Statistics (2001). Participation in Adult Education (Table 359). Washington, DC: U.S. Department of Education. Retrieved December 18, 2003, from http://nces.ed.gov/programs/digest/d01/dt359.asp.

National Hospice and Palliative Care Organization (n.d.). Retrieved June 21, 2006, from http://nhpco.org.

National Institute of Mental Health (2003). *In Harm's Way: Suicide in America* (NIH Publication No. 03-45594). Washington, DC: U.S. Department of Health and Human Services. Retrieved December 16, 2003, from http://www.nimh.nih.gov/publicat/harmaway.cfm.

National Institutes of Health (1991, November 6). NIH Panel Urges Better Management of Depression for Older Americans. *News and Upcoming Activities. NIH Consensus Development Program.* Washington, DC: NIH Office of Medical Applications of Research. Retrieved December 26, 2003, from http http:// consensus.nih.gov/news/releases/086_release.htm.

Newman, K. (2003). *A Different Shade of Gray: Midlife and Beyond in the Inner City.* New York: New Press.

Noel, B., & Blair, P. (2002, February-March). Surviving the Loss of a Partner. *Griefnet.Org.* Retrieved December 26, 2003, from http://griefnet.org/newsletter/febmarsec1.html#losspartner.

Norman, M. (1996, January 14). "Living too long." *The New York Times Magazine,* 36-38.

Nouwen, H.J.M. (1985). *Our Greatest Gift. A Meditation on Dying and Caring.* San Francisco: HarperSanFrancisco.

Nugent, C. (1994). *Mysticism, Death, and Dying.* Albany, NY: State University of New York.

Nussbaum, P.D. (2001). Do brain studies point the way to a "learning vaccine"? *Aging Today, 22,* 1, 17.

O'Connor, E. (1987). *Cry Pain, Cry Hope: Thresholds to Purpose.* Waco, TX: Word Books.

Older Americans 2000: Key Indicators of Well Being (2000). Washington, DC: Federal Interagency Forum on Aging-Related Statistics. Retrieved September 1, 2002, from http://www.agingstats.gov.

Ong, A.D., & Allaire, J.C. (2005). Cardiovascular intraindividual variability in later life: The influence of social connectedness and positive emotions. *Psychology and Aging, 20*(3), 476-485.

Ostir, G.V., Ottenbacher, K.J., & Markides, K.S. (2004). Onset of frailty in older adults and the protective role of positive affect. *Psychology and Aging, 19*(3), 402-408.

Partnership for Caring (n.d.). Washington, DC. Retrieved December 26, 2003, from http://www.partnershipforcaring.org.

Peck, R. (1956). Psychological Developments in the Second Half of Life. In J.E. Anderson (Ed.), *Psychological Aspects of Aging* (pp. 42-53). Washington, DC: American Psychological Association.

Perry, D. (2001). Results of Web-Based "Great Expectations" Survey. *Great Expectations: Americans' Views on Aging.* Retrieved December 26, 2003, from http://www.agingresearch.org/living_longer/summer01/main.html.

Pierson, C. (2000). Issues in End-of-Life Decision Making in the Hospital and Nursing Home Culture. In K. Braun, J. Pietsch, & P. Blanchette (Eds.), *Cultural Issues in End-of-Life Decision Making* (pp. 231-248). Thousand Oaks, CA: Sage.

Pipher, M. (1999). *Another Country: Navigating the Emotional Terrain of Our Elders.* New York: Riverhead.

Polivka, L. (2005, August). The ethics and politics of caregiving. *The Gerontologist, 45*(4), 557-561.

Profile of Informal and Family Caregivers (n.d.). *CareGuide: Care for Caregivers.* Retrieved December 22, 2003, from http://www.careguide.com/Careguide/careforcaregiverscontentview.jsp.

Quinn, J.F. (2001). Retirement trends and patterns among older American workers. *North American Actuarial Journal, 5*(1), 125-126.

Rank, M.R., & Hirschl, T.A. (1999). Estimating the proportion of Americans ever experiencing poverty during their elderly years. *Journal of Gerontology: Social Sciences, 548*(3), S184-S193.

Rappaport, A.M. (2001). Setting the stage: An overview of the retirement 2000 issues. *North American Actuarial Journal, 5*(1), 1-11.

Robert Wood Johnson Foundation (2006). *How Much Does It Hurt?* (Originally published on http://www.lastacts.org). Retrieved February 20, 2006, from http://www.rwjf.org/newsroom/fetureDetail.jsp?featureID=890&type=3&print=true.

Rosenblatt, R.A. (2006, January-February). New report: Social security indispensable. *Aging Today, 27*(1), 2.

Rowe, J.W., & Kahn, R.L. (1987, July 10). Human aging: Usual and successful. *Science, 237*(4811), 143-149.

Rowe, J.W., & Kahn, R.L. (1998). *Successful Aging.* New York: Pantheon.

Rudinger, G., & Thomae, H. (1990). The Bonn Longitudinal Study of Aging: Coping, Life Adjustment, and Life Satisfaction. In P. Baltes & M. Baltes (Eds.), *Successful Aging: Perspectives from the Behavioral Sciences* (pp. 265-292). Cambridge: Press Syndicate of the University of Cambridge.

Ryff, C.D., Magee, W.J., Kling, K.C., & Wing, E.H. (1999). *Forging Macro-Micro Linkages in the Study of Psychological Well-Being.* In C.D. Ryff & V.W. Marshall (Eds.), *The Self and Society in Aging Processes* (pp. 247-278). New York: Springer.

Sarton, M. (1978). *A Reckoning.* New York: Norton.

Schaie, K.W. (1994). The course of adult intellectual development. *American Psychologist, 49*, 304-313.

Schlossberg, N. (1977). The Case for Counseling Adults. In N.K. Schlossberg & A.D. Entine (Eds.), *Counseling Adults. Monterey* (pp. 77-86). Monterey, CA: Brooks/Cole.

Schlossberg, N. (2004). *Retire Smart, Retire Happy: Finding Your True Path in Life.* Washington, DC: American Psychological Association.

Scott-Maxwell, F. (1968). *The Measure of My Days.* New York: Knopf.

Seaver, A.M.H. (1994, June 27). My world now. *Newsweek,* 11.

SeniorNavigator (n.d.). Richmond, VA: Virginia's Resource for Health and Aging. Retrieved May 30, 2006, from http://www.seniornavigator.com.

Seven "secrets" to healthy aging (1999, Spring). *Alliance for Aging Research Newsletter. Living Longer and Loving It.* Retrieved May 30, 2006, from www.agingresearch.org/living_longer/spring_99/feature.htm.

Sheehy, G. (1995). *New Passages: Mapping Your Life Across Time.* New York: Random House.

Simmons, H.C. (1990). Countering Cultural Metaphors of Aging. In J. Seeber (Ed.), *Spiritual Maturity in the Later Years* (pp. 153-166). Binghamton, NY: The Haworth Press.

Simmons, H.C., & MacBean, E.C. (2000). *Thriving After 55: Your Guide to Fully Living the Rest of Your Life.* Richmond, VA: Prime Press.

Simmons, T., & Dye, J.L. (2003). *Grandparents Living with Grandchildren: 2000* (Census 2000 Brief). Washington, DC: U.S. Department of Commerce, Economics and Statistics Administration.

Skinner, B.F., & Vaughan, M.E. (1983). *Enjoy Old Age: A Program of Self-Management.* New York: Norton.

Social Security Administration (2003). *Income of the Aged Chartbook, 2001.* Retrieved January 18, 2005, from http://www.ssa.gov/policy/docs/chartbooks/income_aged/2001/index.html.

Social Security Administration (2006). *Social Security Basic Facts.* Baltimore, MD: Social Security Administration Press Office. Retrieved May 2, 2006, from http://www.ssa.gov/pressoffice/basicfact.htm.

Sonnenfeld, J. (1988). *The Hero's Farewell: What Happens When CEOs Retire.* New York: Oxford.

Stedman, N. (2002, May). A father's death; A daughter's legacy. *Health,* 130-133, 154, 156.

Stoller, E.P., & Gibson, R.C. (2000). *Worlds of Difference: Inequality in the Aging Experience* (3rd ed.). Thousand Oaks, CA: Pine Forge.

Stowe, P. (1996). *Statistics in Brief: Forty Percent of Adults Participate in Adult Education Activities.* Addendum. Washington, DC: U.S. Department of Education, Office of Educational Research and Improvement.

Teilhard de Chardin, P. (1960). *Divine Milieu: An Essay on the Interior Life.* New York: Harper and Row.

Terkel, S. (1995). *Coming of Age: The Story of Our Century by Those Who've Lived It.* New York: New Press.

Thomas, D. (1945). Do Not Go Gentle into That Good Night. In D. Jones (Ed.), *The Poems of Dylan Thomas* (p. 207). New York: Norton.

Thomas, D. (1995, Fall). Age before beauty. *The New York Times Magazine* (Part 2), 22, 24.

Thomas, W.H. (2004). *What Are Old People For? How Elders Will Save the World.* Acton, MA: VanderWyk & Burnham.

Tisdell, E.J. (2003). *Exploring Spirituality and Culture in Adult and Higher Education.* San Francisco, CA: Jossey-Bass.

Tournier, P. (1983). *Creative Suffering.* San Francisco: Harper and Row.

Trelease, M. (1975). Dying Among Alaskan Indians: A Matter of Choice. In E. Kübler-Ross (Ed.), *Death: The Final Stage of Growth* (pp. 33-43). Englewood Cliffs, NJ: Prentice Hall.

Troll, L.C., Miller, S.J., & Atchley, R.C. (1979). *Families in Later Life.* Belmont, CA: Wadsworth.

Troll, L.E. (1982). *Continuations: Adult Development and Aging.* Monterey, CA: Brooks/Cole.

Troll, L.E. (2002). One elder's voice: Living alone—It all depends. *Aging Today,* 23(3), 9.

Trubshaw, R. (1995). The metaphors and rituals of place and time. *At the Edge.* Retrieved January 26, 2001, from http://www.indigogroup.co.uk/edge/liminal.htm.

Uchitelle, L. (2001, June 26). Lacking pensions, older divorced women remain at work. *New York Times,* A1.

U.S. Census Bureau (2000a). *Census 2000 Summary File 3* (Sample Data). Retrieved October 31, 2003, from http://factfinder.census.gov/servlet/DTTable?_ts=8566 7333453.

U.S. Census Bureau (2000b). *Current Population Survey, 2000.* Washington, DC: U.S. Government Printing Office.

U.S. Census Bureau (2001a). *Current Population Report, March 2000* (P20-537). Retrieved June 16, 2006, from http://www.census.gov/population/www/socdemo/nh-fam/p20-537_00.html.

U.S. Census Bureau (2001b). *Statistical Abstract of the United States: 2001.* Washington, DC: U.S. Government Printing Office.

U.S. Census Bureau (2003a). *Current Population Survey, March 2002* (Table 16). Retrieved May 12, 2006, from http://www.census.gov/population/socdemo/race/black/ppl-164/tab16.pdf.

U.S. Census Bureau (2003b). *Grandparents Living with Grandchildren: 2000* (Census 2000 Brief). Washington, DC: U.S. Department of Commerce. Retrieved June 16, 2006, from http://www.census.gov/prod/2003pubs/c2kbr-31.pdf.

U.S. Census Bureau (2003c). *The Older Population in the United States: March 2002.* Washington, DC: U.S. Government Printing Office.

U.S. Department of Commerce (1953). *Statistical Abstract of the United States, 1953.* Washington, DC: U.S. Government Printing Office.

U.S. Department of Commerce (1996). *Statistical Abstract of the United States, 1996.* Washington, DC: U.S. Government Printing Office.

U.S. Department of Health and Human Services (2002, September 16). *National Vital Statistics Report, 50.* Hyattsville, MD: Centers for Disease Control and Prevention, National Center for Health Statistics.

U.S. Department of Health and Human Services (n.d.). *At a Glance—Suicide Among the Elderly.* Washington, DC: National Strategy for Suicide Prevention. Retrieved December 25, 2003, from http://www.mentalhealth.org/suicideprevention/elderly.asp.

U.S. Department of Health and Human Services (n.d.). Medicare. *The Official U.S. Government Site for People with Medicare.* Retrieved December 26, 2003, from http://wwww.medicare.gov.

U.S. House of Representatives (2000). *2000 Green Book.* Washington, DC: Government Printing Office.

Utz, R.L. (2002, November). *The Economic Consequences of Widowhood: How Do Economic Resources Affect Psychological Well-Being?* Paper presented at the meeting of the Gerontological Society of America, Boston, MA.

Utz, R.L., Carr, D., Nesse, R., & Wortman, C.B. (2002, August). The effect of widowhood on older adults' social participation: An evaluation of activity, disengagement, and continuity theories. *The Gerontologist, 42*(4), 522-533.

Vaillant, G.E. (2002). *Aging Well: Surprising Guideposts to a Happier Life.* Boston: Little, Brown.

Verbrugge, L.M., & Jette, A.M. (1994, January). The disablement process. *Social Science and Medicine, 38*(1), 1-14.

Walker, A.J., Manoogian-O'Dell, M., McGraw, L.A., & White, D.L.G. (2001). *Families in Later Life: Connections and Transitions.* Thousand Oaks, CA: Pine Forge.

Walsh, M.W. (2001, Feburary 26). Reversing decades-long trend, Americans retiring later in life. *New York Times,* A1.

Webster, J.D., & Young, R.A. (1988). Process variables of the life review: Counseling implications. *International Journal of Aging and Human Development, 26*(4), 315-323.

Weiss, R. (2005). *The Experience of Retirement.* Ithaca, NY: ILR Press.

Wenger, N.S., Solomon, D.H., Roth, C.P., MacLean, C.H., Saliba, D., Kamberg, C.J. et al. (2003, November 4). The quality of medical care provided to vulnerable community-dwelling older patients. *Annals of Internal Medicine, 139*(9), 740-747.

Whitman, D., & Purcell, P. (2005). *Topics in Aging: Income and Poverty Among Older Americans in 2004* (RL32697). Washington, DC: Congressional Research Service. Retrieved April 3, 2006, from http://digitalcommons.ilr.cornell.edu/crs/1.

Yungblut, John. (1990). *On Hallowing One's Diminishments.* Wallingford, PA: Pendle Hill.

Index

A Journey Called Aging: Challenges and Opportunities in Older Adulthood
© 2007 by The Haworth Press, Taylor & Francis Group. All rights reserved.
doi:10.1300/5915_12